Individuality
in Pain and Suffering

Individuality in Pain and Suffering

Second Edition

Asenath Petrie

The University of Chicago Press
CHICAGO & LONDON

TO
Edwin G. Boring
AND
Ruth S. Tolman
who introduced me
to the generous spirit
of the best Americans

My affiliation with Harvard Medical School and Beth Israel Hospital in Boston and the opportunity of doing a large portion of my work at the Boston Sanatorium (now the Mattapan Chronic Disease Hospital) are among my great privileges. I deeply appreciate the help I received from these three institutions.

The University of Chicago Press, Chicago 60637
The University of Chicago Press, Ltd., London
© 1967, 1978 by Asenath Petrie
All rights reserved. Published 1967
Phoenix Edition 1978
Printed in the United States of America
82 81 80 79 78   9 8 7 6 5 4 3 2 1
ISBN: 0-226-66347-7
LCN: 77-93608

INTERNATIONAL CHRISTIAN
GRADUATE UNIVERSITY

BF
Contents *789*

16813

Figures

Tables

Preface to the Second Edition

How many things by season season'd are.
SHAKESPEARE

It is close to twenty years since I introduced the concept of the neurobiological dimension of reduction and augmentation with sufficient experimental underpinnings to have the communication published in *Science* (1958). "Not all facts are fertile," wrote Edwin G. Boring. I am grateful for the degree of fertility that has resulted in the second edition of this book. My intention is, nevertheless, to try to transcend that accumulation of data to deal with matters that concern me more deeply. I wish to share with the reader some of my thinking on individuality in compassion and callousness which has grown out of the findings about reduction and augmentation.

Before that, let me touch on how these ideas evolved in the first place. As a result of the inquiries received, it is clear that readers are as much interested in this aspect as they are in the present direction of development. The origin of these principles was my research in brain function. Later, I became preoccupied with why certain brain operations gave relief to some patients with chronic pain. After extensive investigations, I became convinced that in these patients the pain remained unaltered, but the associated suffering was nevertheless diminished.

At a symposium (Recent Advances in Neurobiology) held in 1956, I suggested how this might happen: "One aspect of the help that a successful prefrontal lobotomy gives a patient with intractable pain might be an increase in underestimating the incoming painful stimuli." On the same occasion I attempted to explain why suffering is more intense for one type of person in the general population than for another. "I would suggest, as an heuristic hypothesis, that he is the wider open to the environment, that the incoming stimuli are cumulative in him, and that he uses less 'gating' mechanism for cutting them off—his rate of adaptation to them is slower."

After the *Science* article about the augmenter's intolerance for pain and tolerance of sensory deprivation, and about the reversed vulnerability of the reducer, this "reactance" continuum was used to explain varied phenomena in the series of reports that followed. "Whatever theory of pain is held, however many types of pain pathways exist, the reduction goes on in the reducer and augmentation in the augmenter, for these processes are central and express the general perceptual characteristics of the individual," was how I phrased the position in 1963.[1]

At the University of California Medical School in San Francisco, during the winter of 1965–66, came the realization that the time had arrived to enlarge our understanding by returning to the original neurological base and exploring neurophysiological manifestations of reduction and augmentation. To this end, some of the people who worked in the neurophysiological laboratory of Dr. E. Callaway and Dr. B. Spilker were trained by me in the perceptual measurement of reactance as described in Appendix A.

I had demonstrated reduction and augmentation on a perceptual level, had shown that reactance worked throughout the organism, and had postulated a central process as the only way to explain the consistency of the findings. Callaway and Spilker, and Buchsbaum with his colleagues, showed, with the help of techniques that had become available, that these variables could also be demonstrated on a neurophysiological level. Callaway reported these findings involving evoked potential (as described in Appendix E) to me in the spring of 1966. I was a consultant at the National Institutes of Health during that period and shared this information immediately with my NIH colleagues who had become interested in this field at about the same time. They found it very exciting. My hope is that in some measure this stimulated the proliferation of subsequent neurophysiological developments.[2]

---

[1] Asenath Petrie, "Perception and Personality," in *Problems in Dynamic Neurology* (Jerusalem: Hebrew University, 1963).

[2] I have explained the problems created by one proposed modification of the method of measuring perceptual reactance in *Perceptual and Motor Skills* 39 (1974): 460–62. By altering a technique somewhat, one can obtain a feeling of ownership. It is understandable, therefore, that people have attempted to introduce variations of the standardized methods described

It seemed desirable to include a survey of reduction and augmentation as demonstrated neurophysiologically as an additional appendix in this new edition. I invited Dr. Monte Buchsbaum, whose productiveness in this area has been considerable, to prepare it. Some compression of all the new material became necessary because of restricted space.[3]

It is now recommended that a two-pronged approach, both perceptual and neurophysiological, be used whenever possible in determining the degree of reduction or augmentation. In this manner, the perceptual approach will be buttressed by the neurophysiological measurements and vice versa. The new appendix will guide the reader to achieve this.

In this book it is shown that, whether one approaches human variation on a perceptual or on a neurophysiological level, there are clearly disparate ways of handling both the internal and external environment.

Under normal conditions, the closer a person is to the augmentation end of the spectrum, the more he augments the sensory environment. In contrast, the nearer he is to the reduction end, the more he reduces the sensory environment.

This "reactance," that characterizes each person, may be altered to some extent under atypical conditions. For example, overstimulation is followed by a temporary adaptation, in the direction of the reduction end of the spectrum.

Individuality in compassion and callousness is referred to more than once in the body of this book. To take but two examples that emphasize contrasted sensitivity:

> As nurses should be able to empathize with suffering from pain, the dearth among them of those who suffer minimally with pain is worthy of more than the passing notice given it here. (page 7)

> Another serious aspect of the reducer's tolerance for pain, in

---

here even to the point where confusion arises as to what is really being measured. The fact of the validity of the standardized perceptual techniques for demonstrating correlations with neurophysiological variables is therefore stressed.

[3]Fortunately review articles have been published before now on findings about the reactance continuum; two such articles are G. E. Barnes, "Individual Differences in Perceptual Reactance," *Canadian Psychological Review* 17, no. 1 (1976), and James Reason, "Intensity of Feeling," *New Society*, no. 395 (April 1970). In addition there are excellent sources of reference such as the Science Citation Index and the Cumulated Index Medicus.

terms of society, is that he cannot empathize adequately with experiences that he does not share. The extreme reducer fails to understand suffering with pain and may inflict it with little compunction. (page 89)

What I dare write now with considerable certainty is that the feeling of compassion is only possible when there is an understanding that suffering exists in the other. Firm evidence is available to demonstrate that reducers, whose experience of suffering with pain is muted, lack concern about inflicting hurt on themselves or others, or about relieving such hurt. [4]

Perhaps the most helpful analogy is that of a color-blind man trampling small red flowers that are starting to bloom between blades of grass. He is, in fact, unable to recognize that which a person with full color vision would be careful to spare.

It is often a long time before the color-blind person realizes that he has this problem. Neither do those around him recognize it. Punishing the color-blind person is useless. What he needs is help in learning to respond to cues other than color. All these aspects are relevant to our understanding of some forms of callous behavior in the reducer. [5]

The augmenter, on the other hand, whose tendency is to drink in whatever light, sound, and meaning is coming from the environment outside, or to turn his attention with equal openness to what is going on inside himself, suffers greatly from pain. He tolerates isolation and restriction of activities well because he augments his limited sensory environment. He is, therefore, unable to empathize fully with the suffering endured by a reducer in isolation and similar circumstances. Indeed, the augmenter will often seek out just such conditions; this makes it harder to convince him of the contrasted reactance of others. People who sense pain acutely and whose compassion for those subjected to it is a natural outcome of this sensitivity, need to learn to encompass in their compassion also those who appear to lack it. Speaking more generally, the absence of

[4] Dr. Jerry A. Solon, now Program Planning Officer for the National Institute on Aging, and Miss Dora Zolotin, former Director of Nursing at Beth Israel Hospital, Boston, were responsible for significant aspects of this research. My hope is that details will be published elsewhere.

[5] It should be noted, moreover, that the exercise of compassion in one who has suffered pain himself is likely to provide an immediate satisfaction, in the imagination, of what this means to the recipient of his kindness. Meagre rewards of this type in return for compassionate behavior are available to the reducer.

compassion is a danger to humanity. Aggression in each one of us is controlled and inhibited by the compassion that accompanies it.

Our society is changing at a breathtaking pace. Families are broken up. Mobility makes for an end even to the continued presence of kind neighbors. To cope with this mobility, we "travel light." Our religious inheritance, with its built-in safeguards against antisocial behavior, is thrown overboard. The social mores are left behind. It may well be that the time has come when a task which our society needs to undertake is the cultivation of compassion. My hope is that understanding the neurobiological differences between the reducer and augmenter will contribute to achieving this goal.

ASENATH PETRIE

achieved in the findings is due to the assistance of an enormous number of people—some dead and others very much alive—who at one time or another made a contribution that enabled the search to proceed and occasionally provided an inspiration that made it seem to surge forward.

It is impossible to thank Dr. Edwin G. Boring, Edgar Pierce Professor of Psychology Emeritus at Harvard University, as I should like to do. Since I came to the United States he has continually encouraged my work and has also acted as my senior consultant. In addition, he has made invaluable suggestions about the presentation of the material.

It gives me much pleasure to express my deep indebtedness to Dr. Jacob Fine, professor of surgery at Harvard Medical School and Beth Israel Hospital, and to Dr. David Sherman, superintendent of Boston Sanatorium. Their unfailing support made much of this work possible. I am also much indebted to Dr. Jack Ewalt, professor of psychiatry, Dr. Howard H. Hiatt, professor of medicine, and Dr. William Silen, professor of surgery—all of Harvard Medical School—and especially to Dr. Lawrence S. Kubie, recently retired from Yale University, and Dr. Warren McCulloch, of the Massachusetts Institute of Technology, for the time and thought they gave to various aspects of this work.

I am grateful to Dr. John Adams, chairman of the Division of Neurological Surgery at the University of California Medical School in San Francisco and to Dr. Ernest R. Hilgard, professor of psychology at Stanford University, and to their staffs for providing the facilities that enabled me to complete this book. At earlier stages the research was helped by the facilities provided through the Institute of Marine Biology at Wood's Hole, Massachusetts.

The work has benefited greatly from the guidance of Dr. David Finney, F.R.S., now professor at Edinburgh University, who was for a period visiting professor of biomathematics at Harvard Medical School. In the earlier stages Dr. Mindel C. Sheps, now professor at Columbia University, contributed materially to the statistical aspects of the research. More recently, Dr. Robert B. Reed, professor of biostatistics at Harvard University, has advised on this phase of the work. I am also indebted to Dr. Philip Solomon, director of psychiatry at Boston City Hospital, for permitting me to examine some of the subjects in his experimental investigations of sensory insufficiency, and to Dr. Roy O. Greep, dean of the Harvard

School of Dental Medicine, for permitting me to examine some of the patients there.

My colleague Dr. Johanna Tabin as well as Mrs. David Riesman have helped me greatly by discussions at every stage of this work, and by their valuable suggestions after reading the book in manuscript form. Parts of the manuscript were also read and helpful suggestions made by Dr. Theodore X. Barber of the Medfield Foundation, Medfield, Massachusetts; Dr. Abraham S. Freedberg, professor of medicine at Harvard Medical School; Dr. Dale Friend, professor of medicine at the Peter Bent Brigham Hospital; Dr. Richard Jenkins, formerly chief of psychiatric research of the Veterans Administration, Washington, D.C.; Dr. Francis J. Kelley, director of psychological research of the Commonwealth of Massachusetts Division of Youth Service; Dr. William S. Schreiber, chief of physical medicine, Beth Israel Hospital, Boston; and Dr. Jerry A. Solon, professor of medical and hospital administration at the University of Pittsburgh, to each of whom I am much indebted.

Irene Wolk, research assistant in this project for a number of years has been responsible for a large part of the statistical analysis and has made many helpful suggestions on this aspect of the work. Taffy Holland and Phoebe Kazdin have been the chief supervisors of the investigations of patients and subjects and have made other exceedingly valuable contributions to the research. This book could not have been written without the wise and generous help of Evelyn Arac, research secretary to the project for many years. The unstinting help of Peggy Dorfman and Shulamith Rubinfien with the demanding task of proofreading is gratefully acknowledged.

The work was begun and some of the hypotheses developed while, with the support of the Rockefeller Foundation, I was working in England. It was continued in the United States where it was supported by the Foundations' Fund for Research in Psychiatry, Harvard Medical School, the Lasker Foundation, and the Leonard Cohen Foundation of Manchester, England, and also by the National Institutes of Health (Grant M-2641). It is with deep gratitude that I acknowledge my indebtedness to these foundations and institutions, without whose help this work could not have been brought to its present level of advancement.

I am grateful for permission to reprint some of the figures and tables previously published in "Pain sensitivity, sensory deprivation, and susceptibility to satiation," *Science* 128 (1958):

1431–33; "The tolerance for pain and for sensory deprivation," *Am. J. Psychol.* 73 (1960): 80–90; "Some psychological aspects of pain and the relief of suffering," *Ann. N.Y. Acad. Sci.* 86 (1960): 13–27; and "The perceptual characteristics of juvenile delinquents," *J. Nervous Mental Disease* 134, No. 5 (1962): 415–21.

ASENATH PETRIE

Harvard Medical School,
Beth Israel Hospital, and
Mattapan Chronic Disease Hospital,
Boston

1 Intense and Subdued Experience

It is not given to one alone to see all that others see.

MOSES MAIMONIDES, physician (1204)

There is nothing in human experience more central than our capacity to feel, and no aspect of this so crucial as our capacity to suffer, perhaps more particularly to suffer from extremes of physical pain. These capacities result from the impact of events and forces on some particulars of our sensory equipment, and involve our ability to act, to respond, to live, in the most intimate and fundamental ways.

How important it is, then, to gain new exact knowledge in this area of human physical and psychological experience. Such knowledge has been largely lacking in the past, and one reason for this may have been the lack of means to investigate the matter—a means that makes the capacity to feel accessible to test and measurement. In this volume I am undertaking to show that such means exist in the fact that human beings differ remarkably in their individual reactions to pain and suffering.

This book describes a series of studies concerning differences between people in terms of their modulation of sensory experience, ranging from the most intense to the most subdued degree. Between these two extremes we have, for convenience, identified three kinds of persons—the reducer, the augmenter, and the moderate—who differ from one another in their ways of processing their experience of the sensory environment. The reducer tends subjectively to *decrease* what is perceived; the augmenter to *increase* what is perceived; the moderate neither to reduce nor to augment what is perceived. In general these perceptual types [1] occupy adjoining positions on a continuous scale as do, for example, men labeled plump, medium, or thin in accordance with their girth. The work described here is concerned with the effect of differences, especially with relation to suffering, in what we call each person's *perceptual reactance.*[2]

The Contrasted Tolerance of Distress in the Reducer and Augmenter

The research that led to this book was originally concerned with only one of the areas of suffering that we shall be discussing— suffering caused by physical pain. I had been puzzled by the observation confirmed by numerous physicians and nurses that the same trauma affected people so variously. It seemed unlikely that these contrasting reactions to pain [3] were based solely on differences in the control demanded by the culture or by the individual himself. The possibility that culture and will power constitute the total explanation of this variation seemed even more improbable when it became clear that a person's tolerance of pain could be permanently increased by surgical methods that altered his personality (Petrie 1952).

The results of the study reported here suggest a neurological or physiological basis for this variation in tolerance of pain. The individual that we have called the reducer is tolerant of pain; the augmenter is intolerant of it.

A major intention of this work is to point out that sensory lack may result in distress and that the suffering associated with sensory lack also varies from person to person. Our work endeavors to

---

[1] In this volume the word *type* means that the reducer and augmenter represent extremes of a continuous variation—as tall versus short. Unlike the analogy of tall and short, however, the contrast between the augmenter and the reducer involves a tendency toward enlarging versus a tendency toward diminishing.

[2] The term *reactance* is used in the physics of circuit theory. There the reactance of a system, although characteristic of itself, can be altered from the outside by changes in such factors as temperature or pressure. The label is intended here to leave open to future research the question of the parts that heredity and environment play in the degree of reduction or augmentation displayed by a particular person.

[3] In this book, Webster's definitions of pain and suffering are used. Pain is "hurt or strong discomfort in some part of the body." Suffering is "the bearing or undergoing of pain, distress or injury."

show that, whereas at one end of the spectrum of sensation lies suffering occasioned by sensory excess—bombardment with sound, light, heat, and the like—at the other there is suffering occasioned by sensory lack. The variation in suffering from sensory lack or sensory excess appears to be dependent on at least three components: (1) The characteristic perceptual reactance of the individual—that is, his tendency to reduce or to augment or to leave unchanged what is being received; (2) the alterations in his characteristic perceptual reactance that follow upon his ingestion of drugs, or his illness, and the like, at a particular time; and (3) the conditions of his environment—that is, how much freedom of movement and other varied sensory input he is allowed.

In the model developed, pain is thought of as an example of excess of sensory stimulation. Suffering caused by lack of sensation is a much more diffuse kind of discomfort. We shall return in a moment to the relationship to reduction and augmentation of these contrasted kinds of discomfort.

The suffering we shall be considering varies from that of the strong, healthy young man who, after a brief period in an iron lung, where his movements and sensations have been greatly restricted, comes out in a state of panic vowing that no money in the world will ever make him go inside again, to that of the equally healthy dental outpatient who feels he could not have borne the very loud noise of the machine being used for another second. Suffering also encompasses the complex predicament of the alcoholic who, seemingly in the process of relieving one problem, finds himself enmeshed in another, as well as that of the juvenile delinquent who, subjected to solitary confinement, burns himself with cigarette ends in an attempt to relieve his distress, for, paradoxically, he will choose "strong discomfort in some part of the body" to relieve suffering.

We must note at the outset that the observed differences that accompany perceptual augmentation as contrasted with perceptual reduction cover numerous other facets of personality that contribute to the individuality of the suffering. The desire for physical activity, for example, is urgent at the reducing end of the modulation spectrum but not at the other; whereas the desire to be alone part of the time characterizes the augmenting rather than the reducing end of this continuum. These contrasting characteristics are specified below.

First, however, we need to consider this process of perceptual reduction and augmentation.[4] It can be demonstrated that a person's experience of the size of an object held between the fingers gradually changes; the reducer feels as if the object has been reduced in size and the augmenter feels as if it has been augmented. The extent of this change in a few minutes is such that a spectacle case, for example, is experienced by the extreme reducer as though it were half its original size, and by the extreme augmenter as though it were half again as large. We have measured this surprising concertina-like effect by obtaining from each person a series of twelve measurements of the amount of alteration in perceived size occurring during a period of five minutes.

On first consideration it may seem incredible that it is possible to identify the reducer and the augmenter by the use of so relatively simple a form of measurement. The subsequent chapters attempt to explain that the augmenter and reducer, however, are displaying basic differences in their methods of perceiving the environment. All we are doing is obtaining a reliable sample of these differences. It is probable that these contrasts could be demonstrated by means of precise measurement over a period of time with other sense modalities in addition to those few that are detailed here.

In practice, the use of judgments of kinesthetic size, which we have developed as a standard measure, has many advantages; for example, every man has already learned to make judgments of size with his fingers. Moreover, it is easier to maintain attention on something held in the hand than it is to keep attention on a sound. Furthermore, the measurement of size offers minimal technical complication, thus permitting the apparatus to be mobile and easy to use.

The techniques that have contributed to these findings are fully described in Appendixes A and B. A brief description of the

---

[4] The research brought together in this volume was first reported in Petrie (1958) and Petrie, Collins, and Solomon (1958, 1960). Some of the thinking and techniques were stimulated by the pioneer perceptual studies of J. J. Gibson (1933 and later) and W. Köhler and H. Wallach (1944 and later) and the subsequent work of Klein and Krech (1952) and Eysenck (1957). Gibson calls these phenomena "adaptation with negative aftereffect." Köhler and some of his followers refer to them as "figural aftereffect." The accumulating findings, however, have directed the present work into a channel so different from theirs that it seemed wiser not to attempt to relate these two approaches but rather to start afresh with the present concepts of reduction and augmentation.

FIGURE I

APPARATUS FOR MEASURING REDUCTION AND AUGMENTATION

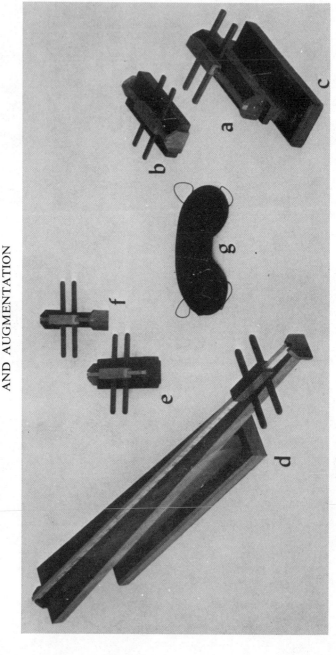

a. 1½ in. Measuring Block. *b.* 2½ in. Stimulating Block *c.* Stand for Stimulating and Measuring Blocks *d.* Tapered Block *e.* 2 in. Measuring Block. *f.* 1 in. Stimulating Block *g.* Blindfold

standardized method for estimating the degree of kinesthetic augmentation or reduction is nevertheless presented here in order that the reader may better follow the argument that leads to the conclusions. In order to use this technique, however, it is essential that the investigator become completely familiar with the detailed instructions in Appendix A.

The Kinesthetic Determination of the Extent of Augmentation and Reduction

Two tests are administered with the equipment illustrated in Figure 1. Both of these tests are given to each subject, but they are separated by a 48-hour interval. The procedures for giving both the tests with the large-block and the small-block stimulation are identical except for the sizes of the rectangular blocks used for stimulation and measurement.

In these tests smooth blocks of unpainted wood are used. In the large-block stimulation test, a block measuring 2½ inches (63.5 mm) in width, is used for stimulation, and a 1½–inch (38.1 mm) block is used for measurement. In the small-block stimulation test, the smallest block, 1 inch in width, is used for stimulation, and the 2-inch block is used for measurement. The block is always held between the fingers of the subject's right hand, unless he is left-handed.

A tapered bar is used to enable the subject to indicate to the tester, with his left hand, the width of the block in his right hand.

The subject is first occupied for 45 minutes without using his hands. Such an empty interval for the hands is essential to allow the effects of previous manual stimulation to wear off as much as possible.[5] Then the subject is blindfolded and feels with the thumb and forefinger of his right hand the width of the measuring block. After that, with the thumb and forefinger of his other hand, he feels the long tapered bar and determines on the bar the place where it

[5] In the situation obtaining in the hospitals and other institutions with facilities to carry out this research, subjects have to be available for meals and other routine events at regular times. The decision that the rest period prior to testing for reduction or augmentation should last 45 minutes is a compromise necessitated by the problems of the institutions cooperating in this study. We have found, however, that after a 15-minute interval following stimulation, scores were, on the average, more than one third of the way back to the prestimulation level (see Figures 2 and 3 and 22 and 23).

seems to be the same width as the measuring block. This measurement is always made four times in succession.

The subject is then given the wider stimulating block to rub with his right thumb and forefinger for 90 seconds. After 90 seconds of rubbing, he is again given the original measuring block and tapered bar and compares them as before, making four separate comparisons.

Next, the rubbing of the stimulating block is repeated for 90 seconds and then for 120 seconds, and four measurements of the subjective size of the measuring block are made after each period of rubbing. After this total of five minutes of rubbing has been completed, the testing is discontinued for 15 minutes. Measurements of the measuring block are repeated after this interval. After an interval of at least 48 hours, the whole procedure is repeated, but on this occasion the stimulating block is narrower than the test block.

The Contrasted Kinesthetic Reactions of the Reducer and the Augmenter

At the end of the period of rubbing, the wooden measuring block is perceived by the extreme augmenter as about 50 per cent increased in size, and by the extreme reducer as 50 per cent decreased in size. The difference between the two thus approaches the size of the object being measured. It may be helpful to think of this phenomenon by considering a sponge that is somewhat compressed to begin with, increasingly compressed for the reducer and allowed to expand to its full size for the augmenter.

When palpation of the block after any of the six periods of stimulation led to a reduction in subjective size of 6 mm or more, we classified the subject as a reducer. If he judged the block as being 6 mm or more larger, we classified him as an augmenter. The other subjects formed the class of moderates. These critical points were chosen because they divided the non-pathological adult population originally studied into three approximately equal groups (see Figures 2, 3, and 4).[6] Figures 5, 6, and 7 show that, on the

---

[6] Later we adopted a slightly more stringent form of classification based on an average of the twelve measurements collected after stimulation during each testing session. When this *average* decreased by 5.4 mm or more, we called the subject a reducer. When the average increased by 5.4 mm or

average, the augmenter enlarges estimated size after stimulation with a block whether the stimulating block is larger or smaller than the block being measured, and that the reverse is true for the reducer, who decreases subjective size in both cases.[7] (See Figures 2 and 4, Appendix C, and the discussion that follows for the degree of correlation between two approaches.) The general tendencies toward augmentation and reduction presented in these graphs have been confirmed in other populations of adults, adolescents, and children—some 570 persons in all (see, for example, Fig. 22 and 23).[8] (Petrie 1960A; Petrie and Collins 1961; Petrie, Collins, and Solomon 1960; Petrie, McCulloch, and Kazdin 1962; Petrie, Holland, and Wolk 1963.)

---

more, we called him an augmenter. This figure of 5.4 is empirically determined as giving reasonably close agreement with the previous classification and so again classifying one-third as augmenters and one-third as reducers. The change was made because of the fear that random variation might play too large a part in using the maximum deviation in estimated size.

The conditions of clinical research necessitated compromise between what is scientifically ideal and what is possible under institutional routine. With patients stimulation usually has to be limited to 300 seconds in spite of the fact that pilot investigations have shown that the reducer, when stimulated for a longer period, will reduce still further, and the augmenter, stimulated longer, will increase his augmentation. This compromise attenuates the difference between those persons who are at opposite ends of the perceptual reactance spectrum.

[7] Included in this population of 156 "normal" persons are some 70 staff and student nurses. What our pilot studies indicate is that nurses who remain in nursing and succeed at it are not usually great reducers. Among this group of 156, the relatively small number of reducers and the excess of moderates seems to be due primarily to the inclusion of the nurses. As nurses should be able to empathize with suffering from pain, the dearth among them of those who suffer minimally with pain is worthy of more than the passing notice given it here.

[8] Among those included in the investigations are some of the outpatients, inpatients, and staff of Beth Israel Hospital (Boston), Boston Sanatorium, and Tewksbury Hospital (office, kitchen, and laundry workers as well as the professional staff); outpatients of the Adolescent Clinic of the Children's Hospital of Harvard Medical School; juvenile delinquents in the Reception Centers of the Commonwealth of Massachusetts; nursing students associated with Beth Israel Hospital (Boston), and University of Pittsburgh Medical School; students of Harvard and Wellesley; students in the Cambridge Public Schools; members of a Roxbury settlement house; young children from the Woods Hole, Massachusetts, and Lincoln, Massachusetts, communities; medical and dental students from Tufts, Northeastern, and Harvard Universities. The sample studied includes a wide range of social and income groups.

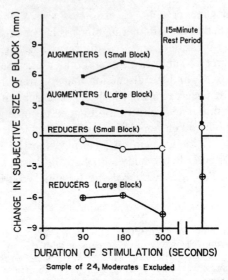

Fig. 2. Reducers and augmenters—stimulation with large and small blocks.

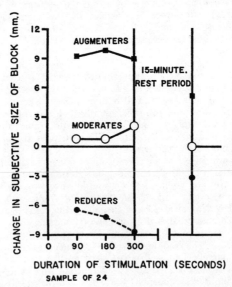

Fig. 3. Reducers and augmenters—stimulation with large and small blocks, combined means.

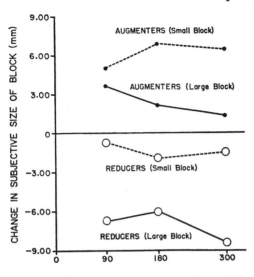

Fig. 4. Effect of stimulation with large and small blocks.

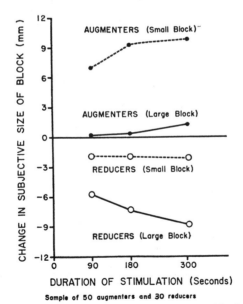

Fig. 5. Effect of stimulation with large and small blocks on 80 augmenters and reducers.

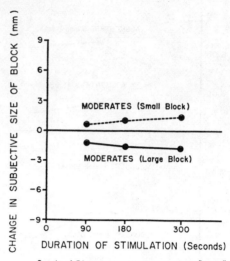

Fig. 6. Effect of stimulation with large and small blocks on 76 moderates.

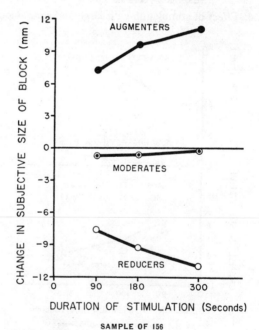

Fig. 7. Effect of stimulation with large and small blocks, combined means.

How the Statistical Results Are Reported

Tests of statistical significance have been carried out on all results presented here. Differences that failed to reach the .05 level of confidence are occasionally mentioned when they are of particular interest but are reported as merely suggestive. All the other findings presented reach at least the .05 level of probability. When they reached the .001 level they were sometimes picked out as being "highly significant." When a difference is in the direction hypothesized, a one-tail test of significance was used.

In general standard statistical techniques have been adequate, such as the t-tests and product-moment correlation coefficients. Analysis of certain critical issues has been reinforced by recourse to non-parametric tests that have, however, always given qualitatively the same conclusions.

Some readers, who will follow the rest of the chapters with ease, may find the statistical section that follows somewhat forbidding. They are urged to move on to the last two paragraphs of this introductory chapter and read on from there. Such selectiveness will not interfere with their understanding of the individuality in pain and suffering.

"Split-Half" Reliability

A type of "split-half" reliability has been calculated using both large-block and small-block stimulation scores of 33 student nurses and 25 public school children. (Details about these persons are given in chapter 5.) The four measurements of equivalent width, made after each of the three periods of stimulation, provided us with 24 difference scores for each subject. For the "split-half" reliability study we correlated the sum of the first and fourth difference scores with the sum of the second and third difference scores. Having arrived at the total degree of augmentation or reduction for each subject during the large-block session on the basis of the first and fourth measurements, we used the same two measurements to calculate the degree of augmentation or reduction during the small-block session and then totaled the values for the small-block and large-block sessions. After that we calculated a second reduction-augmentation score for each person, on the basis of the second and third measurements and followed the same procedure of totaling the values for the small- and large-block sessions. The correlation of these two augmentation-reduction scores yielded an r of .979 for the school children and an r of .973 for the student nurses.

Correlation between Stimulations by Large and Small Blocks

The mistaken notion is prevalent that what is being measured is susceptibility to contrast effects, so that people who show reduction with large-block stimulation will be those who will show augmentation with small-block stimulation. The present hypothesis about the consistency of perceptual modulation proposes that this is not the case. It is of course true that the contrast effect of the smaller stimulus tends to encourage augmentation and inhibit reduction, whereas the larger stimulus encourages reduction and inhibits augmentation. Nevertheless, it appears that the tendency toward augmentation in an augmenter is sufficiently strong to mitigate the contrast effect, and the same relation holds true for the reduction of a reducer.[9]

In a study of 28 adults who were given both large-block and small-block stimulation with a minimum of 48 hours intervening, the correlation of the average change after large-block stimulation with that after small-block stimulation was .767 significant at a probability of 0.0005 (one–tail test).[10]

The frequency distributions of this group are presented in Tables 1 and 2.

The age of these subjects ranged from 23 to 57, the average age being 35.5 years; 23 were females and 5 were males. They came

---

[9] Exceptions are, of course, the atypical stimulus-governed persons described in chapter 5, who appear to respond primarily to the contrast effects. This atypical perceptual reactance occurs in adults with known abnormalities of the nervous system and was also found in some 17 per cent of juvenile delinquents.

[10] It is reported elsewhere that an alteration in perceptual reactance follows upon the ingestion of certain drugs, prolonged sensory stimulation, and also upon an increase in fatigue. This group of 28 right-handed adults consists of persons who, on both occasions of testing were, to the best of our knowledge, free of sickness and other conditions known to cause a change in perceptual reactance.

TABLE 1

FREQUENCY DISTRIBUTION OF LARGE-BLOCK STIMULATION
SCORES FOR ADULT SUBJECTS

Change in Subjective Size of Block (mm)	Number of Subjects
+9.00 or more	0
+7.20 to +8.99	0
+5.40 to +7.19	1
+3.60 to +5.39	1
+1.80 to +3.59	4
0.00 to +1.79	3
−1.79 to 0.00	5
−3.59 to −1.80	2
−5.39 to −3.60	3
−7.19 to −5.40	3
−8.99 to −7.20	2
−9.00 or less	4

TABLE 2

FREQUENCY DISTRIBUTION OF SMALL-BLOCK STIMULATION
SCORES FOR ADULT SUBJECTS

Change in Subjective Size of Block (mm)	Number of Subjects
+9.00 or more	5
+7.20 to +8.99	2
+5.40 to +7.19	0
+3.60 to +5.39	3
+1.80 to +3.59	1
0.00 to +1.79	5
−1.79 to 0.00	5
−3.59 to −1.80	2
−5.39 to −3.60	4
−7.19 to −5.40	1
−8.99 to −7.20	0
−9.00 or less	0

In Tables 1 and 2: $N = 28$; age range $= 23$–57; average age $= 35.5$ (23 female and 5 male).

from among staff and patients at Boston Sanatorium, Beth Israel Hospital and Harvard School of Dental Medicine.

Some further correlations related to the reliability of the methods of measurement are presented in Appendix C.[11]

[11] I am indebted to Thelma Alper, professor of psychology at Wellesley College, to Howard A. and Edward D. Frank, assistant professors of surgery at Harvard Medical School and Beth Israel Hospital, to Celia Sullivan, supervisor of nursing at the Boston Sanatorium, to Jerry A. Solon, profes-

Simpler and Cruder Techniques

It is possible to show augmentation and reduction by simply obtaining finger marks showing the estimated width in a plate of salt, or for more permanent records using finger marks on paper. With this method the precision is less than is obtained with the tapered block so that the method is not to be recommended for anything more than a demonstration, but see Figure 8.

The Modalities in Which Reduction and Augmentation Occur

The various findings in the account that follows and the various modalities in which perceptual modulation occurs suggest that kinesthetic reduction and augmentation, as measured by the standard test, are not independent aspects of perception but are related to input and behavior in other modalities.[12] Indeed, what is being

---

sor of medical and hospital administration at the University of Pittsburgh's School of Public Health and to Miss Dora E. Zolotin, director of nursing at Beth Israel Hospital, Boston, for the studies they instituted and for their generous guidance. Celina Cassels, Ruth Goodman, Peggy Pressman and Everett Jackson, among others, have given great assistance in carrying out some of the testing and computations. Mike H. Lipsky kindly prepared most of the figures.

[12] This evidence is described in detail in the pages that follow. The reader, however, may find it helpful at this stage to survey briefly the modalities in which characteristic perceptual reactance has been shown.

I have already described the method of demonstrating the augmentation or reduction of the perception of size of an object held between the fingers for a few minutes. A pilot study (detailed in Appendix B) has shown that a comparison of augmentation or reduction in the kinesthetic perception of the size of objects, with augmentation or reduction in the perception of the weight of objects, yields a statistically significant relationship.

Some evidence is also presented of the augmentation of light intensities (chapter 2).

There is increased kinesthetic reduction following upon auditory stimulation and thermal stimulation (chapter 4). In addition, it now appears that those born deaf and therefore lacking auditory stimulation, show accentuated kinesthetic augmentation in comparison with those born with normal hearing (chapter 4).

Since a person in a state of reduction is the most tolerant of many types of physical pain, he behaves as if perceptual reactance also affects his perception of pain. In addition, his intolerance of the diminution of sensory supply implies that he is vulnerable to the lessening of the total sensory input from all modalities. (See chapters 2 and 5.)

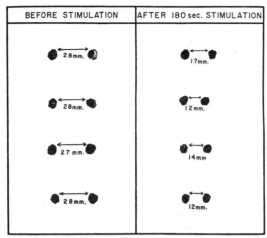

a. Reducer

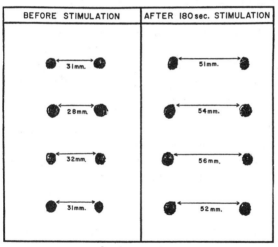

b. Augmenter

Fig. 8. (*a*) The width-judging finger marks of a reducer; (*b*) The width-judging finger marks of an augmenter.

measured kinesthetically seems to be but one aspect of the generalized tendency for the reducer to diminish the perception of stimulation and for the augmenter to enlarge it—two contrasting processes manifesting themselves in different perceptual types in conjunction with other differing characteristics, and particularly with differences in vulnerability.

The Impact of Perceptual
2 Modulation on Suffering from
Pain or from Sensory Lack

To each his sufferings; all are men. THOMAS GRAY (1716)

Individual Variation in the Tolerance for Pain

Varied reactions to physical pain have long been noted by physicians, nurses, and investigators. There is a tendency to assume that these variations are due to differences in the response to an identical experience. The findings on the relationship between tolerance for pain and perceptual reduction or augmentation make it more probable that sensitivity to pain may vary in degree so that some people sense pain acutely, some dimly, and some scarcely feel it at all.

The results of experiments reported in this volume show that the greatest tolerance for pain is shown by a person at the reduction end of the spectrum. It seems that this tolerance for pain is partially due to the tendency to reduce the effectiveness of stimulation. Indeed, the experiments on perceptual reactance described in chapter 1 indicate that this diminution is a cumulative process that persists much longer than the stimulus that initiates the reduction.

A Drastic Alteration in the Patient's Tolerance for Pain

My initial observations were made on patients with pain from incurable conditions that could not be treated successfully by any alternative method—the dose of morphine, for example, could no longer be increased. On occasion such patients were subjected to surgery in the prefrontal region of the brain. I studied a number of these patients before and after such brain surgery.

Surgery in the prefrontal areas of the brain increases tolerance for pain to such a degree that the patient can sleep without morphine and wake without moaning. What is remarkable about this surgery is that it does not deal with the source of the pain; instead, the person himself is changed. The change in personality following brain surgery, measured on a number of different traits, is quite specific when the surgery achieves this effect on pain, as earlier work with some 100 patients has demonstrated (Petrie 1952). Not only is the constellation of personality changes consistent after such surgery, it is more pronounced after a larger than after a smaller incision, it is more apparent when the dominant half of the brain is involved than when the incision is made in the non-dominant half, and it shows less variation in the amount of change when an open operation is performed than when blind surgery is performed.

In contrast, surgical operations outside the prefrontal regions, in the cingulate or temporal areas of the brain, which have no effect on pain sensitivity, are followed by a quite different constellation of personality changes (Petrie 1958).

The implication that certain specific personality characteristics are related to greater tolerance for pain and that these specific characteristics may provide explanatory concepts for such tolerance had begun to concern me earlier (Petrie 1952). Numerous additional factors, as well as the observation of many different kinds of patients, led me to seek evidence of the individuality of suffering—of intense and subdued experience in different persons, and in the same person after treatments that increased tolerance for pain—and thus to the concepts of reduction and augmentation (Petrie 1958, Petrie, Collins, and Solomon 1958).[1]

Experimental Studies of Variation in Tolerance for Pain and Reduction and Augmentation

In the first study, carried out at Harvard Medical School, of variation in tolerance for pain in relation to perceptual reactance,

[1] Eysenck and Nichol's investigations (1958) showing that susceptibility to "figural after-effect" was positively related to extraversion, and the report of Klein and Krech's finding (1952) that certain brain lesions were followed by increased "figural after-effect," combined with the earlier pioneer perceptual studies of J. J. Gibson (1933 and later) and Köhler and his associates (1944 and later) contributed to the initiation of these ideas.

nineteen subjects, paid on an hourly basis, were employed. Pain was induced by the application of heat. The thresholds for pain of these subjects had been determined by Ulric Neisser (Neisser 1959) using an adaptation of the Hardy-Wolff-Goodell dolorimeter, an instrument that concentrates radiant heat upon the skin (Hardy, Wolff, and Goodell 1952). The measurements are of temperature with the higher temperatures arising from longer exposure to the stimulus. The temperature at which the subject first sensed pricking pain was ascertained.[2] Subsequently, the point at which he could no longer endure the pain was determined, the subject being instructed to endure the pain as long as he possibly could. The difference between these two thresholds was used as a measure of the subject's algesic tolerance, a measure that we may call *tolerance for pain*. The distribution of scores measuring their tolerance approximated a gaussian curve. The subjects were divided into groups of low, medium, and high tolerance for pain.

In the determination of reduction and augmentation, the large-block stimulation described earlier was employed. The subjects varied in their perceptual reactance and it was found that those whose perceptual behavior led us to call them augmenters tolerated pain least while the reducers tolerated it best (Petrie, Collins, and Solomon 1958) (See Fig. 9).

The differences in reduction in the kinesthetic task between those with less and those with greater tolerance for pain reached the 5 per cent level of confidence after only 90 seconds of kinesthetic stimulation (see Table 3). Poser (1960) of McGill University has confirmed these observations using pressure as a stimulus for experimental pain and large-block stimulation.

More recently, Ryan and Kovacic (1966) and Ryan and Foster (1966) have demonstrated that highly significant differences in the tolerance of experimental pain are found in comparing those who display most and those who display least perceptual reduction. Using the large-block stimulation test on a group of 60 male high school students, they contrasted 15 subjects who showed the least reduction with 15 who showed the most reduction on two measures

---

[2] The subject's threshold for pricking pain was ascertained at two different sessions, on separate days, and two areas of the skin of the forearm were used during each session. The average of these measurements was used. I was concerned with a threshold of relative constancy, not an absolute one. Some doubt has been voiced about the latter.

)f pain tolerance. The pronounced reducers showed greater pain
tolerance on each occasion, the significance of the difference reach-
ing the .0005 level of probability. The Product-moment correlation
between pain tolerance and the degree of reduction for the group
of 60 subjects reached the .01 level of probability on each occasion.[3]

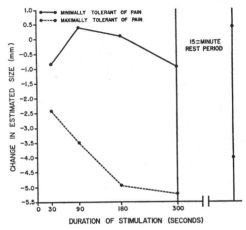

Fig. 9. Comparison of subjects most and least tolerant of pain.

[3] These findings on the relation between tolerance for pain and degree of
reduction are of additional interest because an alteration was introduced
into the method of measuring perceptual reduction. The subject's hand was
alternately placed on the wide or narrow part of the tapered block after
each estimate that he made. It will be noted that the standardized technique
described in this volume is designed to provide minimum changing stimulation for the hand on the tapered block (see Appendix D). To avoid such
stimulation the measurement is always made from the narrow to the wide
section of the tapered block. It is therefore of considerable interest that the
correlation found between pain tolerance and reduction in the standardized
approach can be shown to be present when the technique is altered in the
manner described above.

The method of measuring pain tolerance in Ryan's investigations is worth
describing in some detail. A single plastic aluminum-tipped football cleat
was secured to a curved fiber plate that fitted the leg. The cleat was placed
against the anterior border of the tibia, midway between the ankle and
the knee. Then the sleeve of a standard clinical blood-pressure apparatus
was used to secure the cleat firmly in place. Cleat pressure against the
tibia was induced by inflating the armlet at a slow, constant rate (approximately 5 mm Hg per sec) until the subject indicated verbally that he
was no longer willing to endure the pain. The data were recorded in mm
Hg.

TABLE 3

REDUCTION IN APPARENT SIZE OF BLOCK FOR FIVE GROUPS OF SUBJECTS
DIFFERING IN TOLERANCE OF PAIN AND OF DEPRIVATION
(mm)

TIME OF TEST	PAIN						DEPRIVATION			
	Least Tolerant (N = 7)		Moderately Tolerant (N = 6)		Most Tolerant (N = 6)		Least Tolerant (N = 4)		Most Tolerant (N = 5)	
	Mean	SE	Mean	SE	Mean	SE	Mean	SE	Mean	SE
After 30 sec stimulation	0.81	1.07	0.42	1.68	2.46	1.47	1.26	0.95	−0.03	0.86
After 90 sec stimulation	−0.42[a]	0.77	1.92	1.69	3.50[a]	1.64	1.74	0.75	−0.12	0.83
After 180 sec stimulation	−0.09[ac]	0.56	2.97	1.81	4.95[a]	1.71	4.77[bc]	1.11	1.86[b]	0.70
After 300 sec stimulation	0.96[ac]	0.87	3.36	1.82	5.28[a]	1.96	4.68[bc]	1.23	2.04[b]	0.63
After 15-min rest	−0.42[ac]	0.46	0.72	1.24	4.02[a]	1.35	2.55[c]	0.69	1.83	1.19

Differences are significant between: [a]least and most tolerant of pain; [b]least and most tolerant of deprivation; and [c]least tolerant of pain and deprivation.

The relationship of tolerance for pain to reduction and augmentation recurs in different contexts throughout this book. These are some of the present findings. (1) Alcohol increases both perceptual reduction and tolerance for pain (chapter 3). (2) So does aspirin (chapter 3). (3) So also does audio-analgesia by the use of white noise (chapter 4). (4) The same relationship occurs for frontal lobotomy. (5) Temporal lobectomy, which does not increase perceptual reduction, however, also fails to increase tolerance for pain (Petrie 1958). (6) The schizophrenic during his illness shows pronounced and prolonged reduction and is remarkably tolerant of pain (chapter 4).

Some Clinical Material Illustrating Reduction and Augmentation in Relation to Tolerance of Pain and Discomfort

Some of the insights were suggested by patients in hospital showing extreme tolerance or intolerance of pain. For example, there was a man with a peptic ulcer who experienced no pain at all from his ailment, and he turned out, according to our tests, to be an extreme reducer (see Fig. 10).

In contrast to him there was the patient with severe pain from a phantom limb. At the Beth Israel Hospital in Boston, phantom-limb pain after the amputation of a limb is usually handled successfully by putting the patient on codeine for one week. The staff were puzzled when a young male patient, after the removal of his foot and ankle, required a synthetic morphine four times a day for six weeks. Figure 11 shows the performance of this patient against the background of the augmenters and reducers in Figure 2 of the previous chapter (as was also done for the graph of the patient with the painless peptic ulcer in Figure 10). As will be noted, the patient's augmentation is so pronounced that it put him at the opposite end of the spectrum to the patient with the painless peptic ulcer. It appears that the prediction of great sensitivity in an extreme augmenter holds for pain of central origin as well as for the sensory pain of peripheral origin.

Another example, among our patients contributing to some of the insights, was a boy (with no other pathology) who experienced strong discomfort from light that was tolerated well by the people

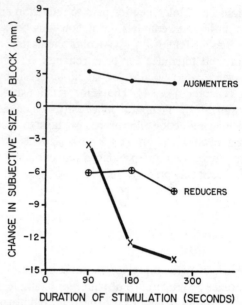

Fig. 10. Male with painless peptic ulcer, effect of stimulation with large block (x———x).

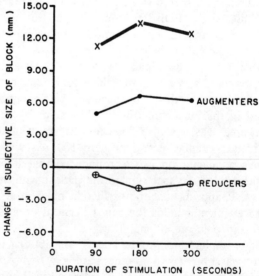

Fig. 11. Male with phantom limb pain, effect of stimulation with small block (x———x).

around him. This patient turned out to show extremely pronounced augmentation (chapter 7 and Fig. 26).[4] In addition, among the dental patients, some of the augmenters experienced great discomfort from the noise associated with audioanalgesia, a noise easily tolerated by the rest of the group (chapter 4). A small study of obstetric patients provided additional supportive evidence of the reducer's tolerance for the pain of childbirth.

Some of the delinquents described in chapter 4 had been tatooed. Since tatooing is painful, we would expect voluntary submission to it to occur in reducers rather than augmenters. That is just what was found: 63 per cent were reducers; 0 per cent were augmenters (significant at .05 level).

The Apprehension of Pain

A burned child does indeed dread fire, but a young child, who has been slightly burned, dreads fire less than one who has been severely burned. It is appropriate to think of the reducer after his experience of the suffering from pain as being a slightly burned child, and of the augmenter as being a badly burned child. Hence the augmenter "fears the fire"—and realistically so—more than does the reducer.

The experiences associated with pain that each person will remember include his sensations and his thoughts about these sensations, as well as the strength of his reactions. Motor memory as well as sensory memory will be different for the two extremes of the perceptual reactance spectrum. The initial simple painful sensation is only briefly present, for the sensations vary in intensity and the cumulative effect of the pain and the associated events presently make the total experience a very complex one. These parts of the total experience exhibit the difference between the reducer and the augmenter, and thus the difference in the apprehensiveness displayed by these two perceptual types when each is confronted with the possibility of further pain. Fear is the augmenter's

---

[4] Some recent findings on the augmentation and reduction of the brightness of light by B. T. Rothman have now been brought to the author's attention. He demonstrated that in a population of 127 normal males (aged 22 to 51) consistent augmentation of the intensity of light occurred in 49 persons and reduction of the intensity of light in 40 persons. A retest reliability study based on a random sample of 30 subjects yielded an r of .783 (B. T. Rothman 1964).

attitude toward pain, as indeed it is toward sensory bombardment in general (Petrie 1960).

Tolerance for Pain and Lack of Preoccupation with Signs of Ill Health

Warning of conditions that may threaten a person's health is provided largely by pain and discomfort. One would predict, therefore, that a preoccupation with symptoms and signs of ill health is less likely to occur in persons who are most tolerant of pain and discomfort. The Minnesota Multiphasic Personality Inventory contains a hypochondriasis scale that explores such preoccupations. J. A. Solon of the University of Pittsburgh School of Public Health, has now shown with some 60 "normal" females that there is a significant negative correlation between the degree of reduction and high scores on the hypochondriasis scale (Solon 1967). Thus, in his population sample, the prediction is borne out that those most tolerant of pain are least preoccupied with signs and symptoms of ill health.

Supporting data comes from a small study conducted by J. Schonfield at the Department of Health in Cambridge, Massachusetts. Among the public school children interviewed, the augmenters were more concerned about particular areas of health than were the reducers (augmenters 55 per cent [$N = 11$]; reducers 9 per cent [$N = 9$]) (Schonfield 1967).

Effect on Behavior of Pathological Conditions Accompanied by Indifference to Pain

Pain, of course, has a protective function. The importance of this function is emphasized in considering the plight of those rare patients born without this protection and who are congenitally indifferent to pain. These persons in early life will sit on hot water pipes until there is a smell of burning flesh and others come to their rescue. They will walk about with broken bones, unaware that anything is amiss and adding greatly to the damage done. Later, in order to survive, they learn to respond to cues other than pain. One patient, a nineteen-year-old student, indifferent to the pain from very hot water, needed to be especially careful to avoid scalding herself and her mother when she was helping to wash dishes (Cohen *et al.* 1955). As children, moreover, these individuals will hurt their fellows in play, for they do not know what "hurt" means. "He jests at scars who never felt a wound."

That intact survival is jeopardized in the absence of pain is reinforced by the effects of certain diseases that may occur quite late in life. For one example, sensitivity to pain is lost in leprosy. Recent workers have demonstrated that many of the problems in treating leprosy arise from the lack of this "danger" signal, and the consequent neglect by the leper of wounds and infection. Among the most bizarre of such reports is that a rat can nibble away at the fingers of a leper who sleeps on with no pain to disturb and protect him.

Tolerance for Pain and Risk of Physical Injury

Since pain has such important protective functions and since the reducer is least sensitive to it and least preoccupied with signs and symptoms of ill health, it seemed reasonable to me to predict that he would be less careful in avoiding painful injuries than would be the augmenter who is most sensitive to pain. Solon has recently shown, with a group of some seventy student nurses that while an equal proportion of reducers and augmenters come to the Health Services for treatment, accidents occurred in 86 per cent of reducers and 46 of augmenters. This difference is highly significant (Solon 1967).

Avoidance of cigarette smoking is a health precaution taken by some persons. We might also predict that smoking would be less pronounced in augmenters than in reducers. It will be seen in chapter 6 that augmenters start to smoke later in life, smoke less, and give up smoking more frequently than reducers.[5]

Some Further Notes on Pain and Reduction and Augmentation

Our findings suggest that the reducer's greater tolerance of pain is independent of the cause of the pain. The processing of the pain is

[5] In connection with augmenters taking precautions to maintain health, another finding from Schonfield's study is of interest. In a very small sample of public school children it was found that augmenters, as compared with reducers, prefer nutritionally valuable foods at breakfast (augmenters = 66 per cent [N = 9], reducers = 0 per cent [N = 5]).

determined by the perceptual reactance of the patient, and the sensations will be reduced by the reducer and augmented by the augmenter.

The more intense experience of the augmenter and his associated greater apprehensiveness of pain and discomfort will have their counterparts in the reactions of his autonomic nervous system. For example, his pulse, his rate of breathing, and the amount he perspires are likely to be affected. Indeed, it is not improbable that many of the items measured on a lie-detector test would differ at the two ends of the perceptual modulation spectrum. The magnitude and frequency of the augmenter's reactions, in contrast to those of the reducer, might easily lead to the mistaken notion that the variations are due to the instability of his nervous system rather than to his perceptual reactance, as this research suggests.

Tolerance for Pain as Distinguished from the Pain Threshold

Tolerance for pain and the pain threshold are frequently and mistakenly considered identical. When pain is induced by gradual increase in heat, for example, the pain threshold is the temperature at which the subject first senses pricking pain. The reducer's greater tolerance for pain does not mean that he necessarily has a higher pain threshold. The total time a subject can endure the stream of sensory bombardment may be a factor more important in tolerance for pain than is the pain threshold. The pain threshold remains unchanged after a prefrontal lobotomy and may also remain constant after pain-relieving drugs, although increased tolerance for pain and increased reduction occur in both cases. A change in pain threshold, therefore, need not accompany increased tolerance for pain, whereas increased perceptual reduction apparently does accompany such increased tolerance. What is suggested here is that the extent of augmentation or reduction is an indication of tolerance of pain.

Perceptual reactance is a process occurring in time. The process can be observed in short periods of time—a matter of a few minutes only—but these moments are essential. We tend to mistakenly assume that a person's perceptions of the same stimuli are constant; in fact, however, these perceptions are modulated over a period of time. Tolerance and intolerance for pain are also processes occurring in time. The inclusion of the dimension of time in our thinking brings into our observations of perceptual behavior some ordered patterning that is otherwise missing.

Contrasted Tolerance for Confinement and Isolation in the Reducer and Augmenter

The greatest tolerance for pain is shown by the person who is perceptually reducing. This tolerance is due in part, it seems, to his tendency to reduce the perceived intensity of stimuli. Thus an intermittent intense wave of pain may cause later pain to appear to him to be less severe.

If the reducer's tolerance of pain is partially due to his tendency to diminish the perception of the stimulation, then this tendency to reduce becomes a handicap in a situation where the environment starves the individual of sensation instead of bombarding him with sensation, as is the case with pain. Such sparsity of sensation occurs, for example, in confinement and isolation in chronic illness. Pronounced disturbance of behavior and of subjective states are frequently associated with persistent conditions of sensory lack. We have now come to recognize that the nervous system needs sensory stimulation almost as much as the digestive system needs nutriment. The ill effects of an acute shortage of sensory input were originally shown at McGill University (Bexton, Heron, and Scott 1954), then were substantiated and detailed by J. C. Lilly (1956), and have since been investigated and repeated in a number of other centers. (A selection of such reports is presented in Solomon *et al.* 1961.)

Experimental and actual sensory deprivation is never complete and is often merely a lack of variety of stimulation. Nevertheless, just as contrast and change are the conditions of attention, so monotony is in fact psychologically the equivalent of diminution in sensory input. In the sensory limitation accompanying confinement and isolation, a strong tendency for the reducer to diminish the perceptual intensity of a sound—after he has heard a louder or softer sound, for example—would make the sum total of sound for him less than for the augmenter. Thus being a reducer should make for intolerance of confinement and isolation because it would render the already limited stimulation even less effective; the reducer would consequently be more troubled by his confinement and isolation.

Experimental Studies of Tolerance for Sparsity of
Sensations and Reduction and Augmentation

Our findings from two different groups of 17 volunteers subjected to sensory deprivation indicate that such a relationship holds. Augmenters tolerate starvation of stimulation and willingly remain in a tank type of respirator longer than do the reducers. This difference is exactly the reverse of the behavior of these two types under the stress of pain.

In the studies of the tolerance of sensory lack the subject was placed on his back in a respirator of the type popularly known as an "iron lung." The vents were left open so that there was no interference with breathing. Through the opening at the top of the respirator the subject could only view the greyish white ceiling. His arms and legs were placed in cardboard cylinders to reduce movement and tactile contact as much as possible. The respirator motor, which produces a monotonous, dull, masking sound, was kept running and thus the observer, who was always present, was out of hearing as well as out of sight.

The subject was paid by the hour and was informed that the research was an attempt to find out how normal, healthy persons responded to being placed in this type of respirator. Each was told that the experiment would be stopped in 36 hours but that he could end it at any time he wished. The length of time he was willing to remain in the respirator was used as the measure of his tolerance.

Results for the first group of nine subjects are given in Figure 12 and Table 3. In the second group of volunteers, the difference in perceptual reactance between the good and poor tolerators of deprivation is significant beyond the 2 per cent level of confidence. Indeed, when the two deprivation groups are combined, the difference in perceptual reactance after 120 seconds of stimulation is significant beyond the 1 per cent level. Thus perceptual reduction can possibly be seen to play a part in the mechanism of the intolerance of sensory deprivation, for it causes the limited stimulation available to be perceived as even less intense. One may think of the reducer as being subjected in his day-to-day life to some sensory scarcity; the greater his tendency to reduce, the greater his sensory lack. He becomes intolerant of further sensory lack. At the other end of the spectrum is the augmenter, whose incoming sensory content is increased by previous perception. His pain and other sensations are undiluted but he tolerates sensory deprivation more readily. In other words, different kinds of resistance are needed for tolerating the stress of pain and the stress of isolation and confinement.

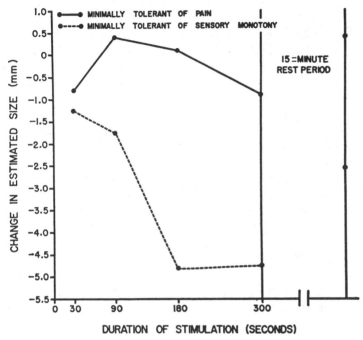

Fig. 12. Comparison of subjects least tolerant of sensory deprivation and least tolerant of pain.

Contrasts in Behavior of Patients during a Period of Restricted Activity and during Childbirth

To extend the findings of the relation of the tolerance for pain to tolerance for restriction of activity and incarceration in a clinical situation, my associates and I studied a small sample of healthy expectant mothers who were kept in the hospital for some months before the birth of their babies, primarily because these babies would be illegitimate. I had a number of items in the behavior of these women assessed by independent judges during the restrictive period prior to labor and during actual childbirth. The assessments lent some support to the earlier findings about the contrasted tolerance for pain and for restriction of activity at the two ends of the perceptual reactance spectrum.

During restriction to the hospital, the women were rated by three judges on a three-point scale with regard to five aspects of their behavior: "multiple complainer," "critical," "poor or lazy worker," "uncooperative," and "trouble-maker." We found six augmenting and moderate and only two reducing mothers whose subsequent labor was classified as normal and comparable. In this group of eight, as well as in a slightly larger one, the ratings indicated that the augmenters and moderates behaved best and the reducers worst during the period of restriction. (The difference was significant at the .01 level.)

The same patients were rated according to their tolerance for the pain of childbirth by two judges independently—the physician in charge and a nurse—who, in coming to their decisions, took into consideration the patients' demands for analgesic drugs, their sleeplessness as said to be caused by pain, their physical signs, and their statements about their experience. The physician and nurse did not know the perceptual reactance scores of these patients and the tester did not know the ratings given. The rating results indicated that the augmenters bore clinical pain least easily. We were able to obtain assessments of two other mothers only on their behavior during labor but, again, they showed that the reducer tolerated the pain of childbirth better.[6]

Reducers Expressed Preference for Pain over Solitary Confinement

Solitary confinement is still practiced in some of the institutions where juvenile delinquents are detained. The boys in one institu-

[6] The work has benefited by help from Walter Collins, now chief, Outpatient Clinic in the department of radiology at Boston City Hospital, particularly in the investigations of patients in pain and the effect of pain-relieving drugs; from Lois Crowell, physician at Tewksbury Hospital, where some of the studies of tolerance of confinement were conducted; and from Ulric Neisser, who, while teaching at Harvard's Department of Psychology, carried out the testing and computations in the experimental study of pain. I am also indebted to Sumner E. Liebman, head of the department of ophthalmology at Beth Israel Hospital, and to E. W. Friedman, instructor in surgery at Harvard Medical School, for their cooperation in the investigations of their patients.

tion in Massachusetts were asked whether they would prefer confinement to pain. Every reducer expressed a preference for pain (see chapter 5).

Contrasted Attitudes to Pain in Relation to Tolerance for Confinement

Contrasting attitudes concerning their pain were, moreover, expressed by subjects most and least tolerant of the stress of experimental sensory lack. These two groups also differed in their estimations of their tolerances for pain, in their opinions of their parents' attitudes toward the expression of suffering with pain, and in their evaluation of the pain they had experienced during isolation in the respirator. Those who were unable to tolerate much deprivation believed themselves able to stand pain especially well and did not believe that the parental demand for self-control in their youth, control in the expression of suffering with pain, had been stringent. On the other hand, those persons who were able to stand sensory deprivation well did not think they could stand pain well and believed that the parental demand for self-control in the expression of suffering with pain had been unduly stringent. Thus, it appears in this group also that he who is least susceptible to deprivation is most susceptible to pain and vice versa.

To examine this generalization further, we decided to seek from the subjects who had undergone experimental deprivation a subjective quantitative estimate of the pain they shared in common—the muscular pain associated with being confined in a respirator. Each of eight subjects was asked what proportion of his earnings from the experiment he would forgo could he be relieved of the pain when required to repeat the rest of the experiment. Of the four subjects who stayed longest in the respirator, one offered to do without 100 per cent of his earnings to avoid the backache. Another offered 50, a third 40, and a fourth said that he had felt discomfort rather than pain and that this had not been an important factor in his experience. Of the four subjects who stayed in the respirator the shortest period, one said he would never undertake the experience again for any amount of money and that the ordeal was infinitely worse than the most agonizing pain he could imagine. Two who said they had abandoned the confinement because of the pain were not ready to forgo any earnings to be relieved of the pain, and one agreed to forgo 25 per cent of his earnings.[7]

It appears that the absence of pain is more greatly valued by those subjects who tolerated sensory lack best. They were the subjects at the augmenting end of the spectrum. Implicit in these findings is the fact that the non-tolerators of sensory lack at the reducing end of the spectrum were much more troubled by other aspects of the experience than by the pain—aspects that constitute the characteristic nature of the stress of sensory deprivation. Perhaps they, nevertheless, complained of pain rather than the other aspects because our culture regards pain as a signal of which it is proper to take notice.

Our language is rich in words for description of pain. The stress of sensory lack, however, has no such richness of expression in our contemporary culture or language. It is of interest that, according to the *Oxford Shorter Dictionary,* about 400 years ago "stress" as a verb meant "to confine or incarcerate."

If it were necessary to explain the sensations of bodily hunger and of the relief that accompanies the cessation of hunger, to a person who had felt neither, it would be difficult to find the appropriate words. To describe the satisfaction accompanying the "end of a lack" is a hard task. Thus the difference in the range from joy to suffering between the augmenter and reducer may possibly lie largely in the latter's inability to describe these states.

Tolerance for Pain and for the Stress of Sensory Scarcity as Related to the Scores on the Maudsley Personality Inventory

The Maudsley Personality Inventory is a brief and reliable measure of two relatively independent broad factors of personality—

[7] In addition to the answers to standardized questions that served to differentiate the attitudes of the reducer from those of the augmenter, as collected from the students, the school children, and others, many persons who turned out to be at the extremes of the reduction-augmentation spectrum made spontaneous comments that suggested some of these personality characteristics. For example, during the test that involved judging the passage of an empty period of time, a reducer said, "I *hate* quiet times"; while a girl at the augmenting end of the spectrum in one of the pregnant groups studied said that she would hesitate to have another baby because of the pain involved.

"neuroticism" and "extraversion-introversion." "Neuroticism"—N —refers to general emotional instability, emotional over-responsiveness and predisposition to neurotic breakdown under stress. "Extraversion"—E—refers to outgoing, uninhibited, impulsive, and sociable inclinations. The method of developing the inventory was factor analytic and is adequately described in the *Manual* (Eysenck 1959, 1962).

The Maudsley Personality Inventory consists of 48 items, of which 24 are keyed to "neuroticism" and 24 to "extraversion-introversion." The manual prepared by Robert Knapp for the American edition has a bibliography of 112 items of the most relevant literature and summarizes many of the published findings (see also Eysenck 1957, 1962). It also presents norms based on 1,064 American university undergraduates. Means and standard deviations are presented for 32 different groups, including various psychiatric, prison, and industrial populations, totaling over 7,000 subjects. Factor-analytically sophisticated readers are also referred to Carrigan's critical appraisal of "Extraversion-Introversion" as a dimension of personality (1960).

Reliability and Validity. "Split-half" and Kudder-Richardson estimates of item intercorrelations for each scale are between .75 and .90 in various samples. Test-retest reliabilities range from .70 to .90.

"Neuroticism" and "introversion-extraversion" scales have high loadings on factors that are also heavily represented in other measures considered to be indicative of neuroticism or extraversion, and there is little factorial overlap between the "neuroticism" and "extraversion-introversion" scales. The "neuroticism" scale correlates with the Taylor Manifest Anxiety Scale. Taylor's Manifest Anxiety Scale, however, has a slightly greater correlation with "extraversion-introversion" than does the "neuroticism" scale.

Descriptive validity of the Maudsley Personality Inventory has been established by the method of nominated groups. Judges rated people on the basis of observable characteristics in terms of neuroticism and extraversion. These ratings show highly significant correlations with the relevant dimensions as measured by the Maudsley Personality Inventory.

Interest in the Maudsley Personality Inventory was due to the author's earlier work with brain lesions. Taken as a whole, the constellation of personality changes after brain operations increasing tolerance for pain shows the patient to be more "extraverted" and less "introverted" after the alteration (Petrie 1952). This is *not* the pattern of personality change with brain operations that do not increase tolerance for pain (Petrie 1958).

Three aspects of the data from the Maudsley Personality Inventory seem particularly interesting. Those persons tolerating experimental pain best showed the higher "extraversion" scores. Those tolerating clinical pain best also showed higher "extraversion" scores. On the other hand, those showing most tolerance for isolation had the lower "extraversion" scores.

This contrast recorded by the Maudsley Personality Inventory parallels the contrast in perceptual reactance, for, it will be remembered, the reducers are most tolerant of pain, and the augmenters most tolerant of isolation.

The Maudsley Personality Inventory was used with five separate groups of patients and subjects, 65 in all, on whom we had pain tolerance measures. The patients had been subjected to major chest surgery, minor surgery, or bronchoscopy. In addition, we used the inventory with volunteers who were subjected to experimental thermal pain and with the first group of volunteers who had been subjected to experimental sensory deprivation.

The patients in this study who were experiencing clinical pain—as in the obstetric group described above—were rated according to their tolerance for pain caused by comparable trauma by three judges independently—a physician, a surgeon, and a nurse. In coming to their decision the judges took into consideration the patients' demands for analgesic drugs, physical signs and statements of patients. These judges did not know the scores of the patients on the other tests. Patients were interviewed by the physician on two occasions while they were in pain. The assessment form used is shown in Figure 13. (The subjects represented the extremes of tolerance and intolerance for pain. Those moderately tolerant of pain were omitted from consideration.)

In all five groups the differences were in the expected direction. The higher "extraversion" scores were found in the best tolerators of pain, while those who were least tolerant had the lowest "extraversion" scores. The relationship is reversed for sensory deprivation; those who tolerate the stress of isolation best have the *lowest* "extraversion" scores. These scores are summarized in Table 4.

The "N" scores in this personality inventory are intended to

	None	Slight	Moderate	Severe	Agony
1 Involuntary verbal expressions of pain (e.g., moaning, yelling, screaming).					
2 Demand for analgesics.					
3 Spontaneous reports of pain.					
4 Restlessness.					
5 Squirming, stiffening, gripping.					
6 Interference with breathing.					
7 Interference with talking.					
8 Physical signs of pain (e.g., blanching, sweating, tremor, dilation of pupils).					
9 Interference with sleeping.					
10 Interference with eating and other daytime activities.					

Fig. 13. Form used to assess pain reactions.

TABLE 4

"EXTRAVERSION" SCORES ON THE MAUDSLEY PERSONALITY INVENTORY FOR FIVE
CLASSES OF SUBJECTS FURTHER DIVIDED INTO SUBGROUPS ON THE BASIS OF
TOLERANCE FOR PAIN AND TOLERANCE FOR SENSORY DEPRIVATION

Class of Stress	N	Most Tolerant Subgroup	Least Tolerant Subgroup	Direction of Difference
Pain from:				
Major chest surgery	16	24.90 *	21.30	+
Minor surgery	9	25.90	18.50	+
Bronchoscopy	17	27.40	26.50	+
Experimental pain	13	28.67	23.57	+
Sensory deprivation	10	28.50	31.80	−

* Higher "Extraversion" scores characterize the patient after lobotomy and the more
psychopathic patient. The difference between subgroups is significant at the 5 per cent
level.

measure the degree of "neuroticism" present. In contrast to the differential findings with the "extraversion" scores, no differences at all were apparent in the "neuroticism" scores in any of the groups studied. Thus "neuroticism" as measured by this inventory does not appear to contribute to the tolerance or intolerance of either the stress of pain or of confinement.

In another adult group of 38 persons in which the Maudsley Personality Inventory and perceptual reactance scores had been obtained, differences between reducers and augmenters in the expected direction were also found.[8] The reducers provided significantly higher extraversion scores than did augmenters (30.0 as against 23.8—.01 probability level). There was again, in this group, no difference in the scores for neuroticism (19.6 and 20.8, respectively).

Conditions That May Diminish the Stress of Sensory Insufficiency

We have found that the reducer is physically more active than the augmenter, thus deriving considerable sensory input from his own body movements (chapter 7). The contrast in physical activity for persons with these differing perceptual styles is particularly relevant when sensory lack is combined with restriction of activity, as is the case in most experimental studies of sensory deprivation. A greater proportion of the reducer's sensory "income" is derived from the sensations of movement than are those of his opposite perceptual type.

The inactive augmenter, on the other hand, excels at schoolwork and there is other evidence that he relies on verbal behavior in becoming related to his environment and for much of his sensory homeostasis (see chapter 7). For this reason, one may not disregard the part that subvocal speech, associated with intense thought, may play in introducing variety into monotony and diminishing sensory lack, particularly in augmenters.

[8] Of the 38 subjects in this group who came from the staff and patients at Boston Sanatorium, Beth Israel Hospital, and Harvard School of Dental Medicine, 16 were females and 22 were males. The age range was 24 to 67 years, the average age being 46 years. There was no appreciable difference in sex or age distribution in comparing reducers with augmenters.

The Choice of Pain

Delinquents at the reducing end of the spectrum, punished with solitary confinement, will frequently carve their own flesh with razors and burn it with cigarette ends. Under the stress of sensory deprivation, physical pain may become for them the lesser of two evils (chapter 5). Such phenomena may be partly accounted for by the fact that while, on the psychological level, the process of habituation to a sensation is accompanied by the nervous system's cutting off monotonous stimulation, pain is not quickly blocked out (Adrian 1928 *a* and *b*), and under ordinary conditions complete habituation for it scarcely occurs. Such non-habituation to pain contributes to the protection of the organism (Dallenbach 1939, Stone and Dallenbach 1934). In sensory monotony or deprivation, the absence of adaptation to pain results in a diminution of the sensory starvation and the pain itself actually provides sensory nourishment. He who is starved of sensation—particularly if he is at the reducing end of the spectrum—may find that pain, as a sensation, constitutes an alleviation of his stress.

Further support to this view is given by the observation that animals brought up in a restricted sensory and social environment behave as though some forms of pain are not noxious. For such animals, the normal avoidance of pain is absent. One chimpanzee had been restricted in tactual, kinesthetic, and manipulative experience during the first 31 months of its rearing. Subsequently when it was pricked with a pin it often responded by panting as chimpanzees do when they are being tickled and enjoying the stimulation (Nissen, Chow, and Semmes 1951). A Scotch terrier that has been reared under conditions of extreme sensory deprivation puts his nose into the flame of a lighted match. This type of behavior does not occur in animals provided with the usual amount of sensation during rearing (Melzack and Scott 1957).[9] It is not impossible that such findings on the attractiveness of pain in sensory starvation may also turn out to have some relation to the origin of masochism in man. For example, extreme perceptual reduction during early youth, in conjunction with an environment

[9] That persons who are born deaf show in adulthood greater agumentation than those born with normal hearing is of interest in this connection (chapter 4), as is the possibility of the conditioning of perceptual reactance (chapter 3).

that fails to provide for the needs created by this characteristic, could conceivably lead to a pathological appetite for sensation.

The Sensory Reduction accompanying Alcoholic and Schizophrenic Hallucinations

The increased reduction of perception following upon the intake of alcohol is described later (chapter 3). We shall see in chapter 5, moreover, that the alcoholic is particularly susceptible to a pronounced change toward the reducing end of the spectrum after he has consumed alcohol. Thus we find that hallucinations due to alcoholism occur under conditions of pronounced reduction of sensory input.[10]

Also relevant to the presence of hallucination when there is a dearth of sensory input are the findings in a study of schizophrenics (chapter 4). During the schizophrenic phase of their illness, the majority of the patients studied appeared to be in a "spasm of reduction"; there was a clamp on sensations received from the environment.

The question arises as to how sensory lack may contribute to the production of hallucinations. Sensory input—what we hear and see and touch—acts as a check on the difference between reality and our fantasies; we pinch ourselves to see if we are awake. It is interesting to hypothesize that diminution of sensory input possibly makes such differentiation more difficult, and for some persons under these conditions their fantasies may become reality.

But the main intent of this chapter is to show that within the normal population, perceptual augmentation and reduction appear to affect the tolerance for pain and for sensory scarcity. This is not to gainsay that other factors also influence such tolerance—factors that have been discussed by , among others, Head (1920), Adrian (1928 a and b), Hebb (1933), Nafe (1934), Boring (1950), Freeman and Watts (1950), Gerard (1951), Weddell (1955), White and Sweet (1955), Lilly (1956), Keele (1957), Beecher (1959), Bishop (1959), Noordenbos (1959), Wolff and Jarvick (1964), and Melzack and Wall (1965). The consistency of the relationship, despite all the other influential factors, between perceptual modulation and the tolerance of pain and stress might be seen as encouraging further research with this approach.

[10] During sleep there is, of course, a pronounced diminution of afferent input—and it is then that the hallucinations we call dreams occur.

Drugs Causing Alterations in
3 Augmentation and Reduction

And men do differ from themselves as well as from other persons. SIR THOMAS BROWNE, physician (1605)

ALCOHOL

Alcohol causes a reduction of suffering in some people; indeed, insofar as physical pain is concerned, it was one of the first anesthetics ever used. There is also the problem of addiction to alcohol. Any light that can be thrown on alterations of personality induced by its consumption and the nature of these alterations may contribute to an understanding of this social and medical problem, as well as to our understanding of suffering.

Our initial hypothesis was that the effect of this drug is partly due to a change in perceptual reactance—a change that is closely related to the tolerance of pain.

The Kinesthetic Reduction Caused by Alcohol

Twenty-seven subjects were employed, members of the staff of the Boston Sanatorium. Among them were kitchen and laundry workers, clerks, nurses, surgeons, and physicians. Teetotalers and persons who had problems with alcohol were excluded from the experiment so as to limit the number of complicating variables in this initial investigation. Seven of the subjects were augmenters, ten were reducers, and ten were moderates. Each subject was told that he was taking part in an investigation into the effect of alcohol and alcohol-like drugs. Each was seen on three occasions. On the first occasion, no drug was administered. We obtained a base line from which to estimate the effect of the procedure introduced on the two remaining occasions, the order of which was randomly arranged. On one of the subsequent occasions, a glass containing grapefruit juice, two ounces of vodka and a straw was given to the subject by a physician and the subject was instructed to drink it through the straw.[1] (Vodka was used as it is relatively tasteless. It was 80-proof, that is, its volume was 40 per cent alcohol.) On the other occasion, the same procedure was followed, but the alcohol was omitted. Each time the patient was warned not to drive immediately after the experiment and to take other precautions that were sensible after the consumption of alcohol. Neither the experimenter, the subject, nor anyone else in contact with them knew when the alcohol had been omitted.

A drug is usually evaluated in the literature by considering its effect on the group studied as a whole. The findings about drugs, therefore, are first presented in this accepted fashion. It will be shown below, however, that important facets of the drug's effectiveness only become apparent when perceptual subgroups are considered separately.

The overall effect of alcohol, comparing it with what may be called the "feigned alcohol," was an increased tendency to reduce. (The changes found after "feigned alcohol" are discussed below.) Thus, one part of the hypothesis is supported: the effect of alcohol in increasing the tolerance for pain and suffering could partially be due to its ability to increase the tendency to reduce and thus to diminish the subjective intensity of perceived pain.

In fact, however, such an overall view hides a much more important finding, for if we break down our population into augmenters, moderates, and reducers, we find that after the consumption of alcohol it is the augmenters in whom the maximum and dramatic change is found, for they cease enlarging and begin to reduce. Diminished augmentation occurred in every one of the augmenters. The average change of the group of augmenters had a P-value of .001. The moderates, however, showed almost no change at all. The reducers changed a little, though not so much as

---

[1] Drinking through a straw enabled the subject to avoid using his hands; this "hand resting" is important for 45 minutes before measures of perceptual reactance are made.

he augmenters; the direction of the change was to make them reduce slightly less [2] (see Figs. 14 and 15 and Table 5).

What all this means is that the consumption of as little as two ounces of alcohol is followed by a most significant increase in reduction in augmenters. It is here suggested that this reduction

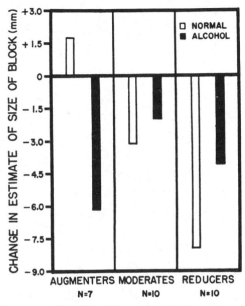

Fig. 14. Effect of alcohol.

[2] Analysis of variance was used with the alcohol results. The scores obtained after each of the periods of stimulation were compared to ascertain the effect of the normal score of alcohol and the "feigned alcohol." The reducers, augmenters, and the moderates were treated separately. In addition to the differences after each period of stimulation, the average effect of the three periods of stimulation was calculated. The bar graph (Fig. 14) presents the mean effect of the alcohol on the tendency of these three groups to reduce.

Changes resulting from alcohol, or any other pain-relieving method, are composed of two parts. The first is the change which would be the result of sampling error; for the extreme groups this would tend to regress the average scores of both augmenters and reducers towards the moderates. The second part, which is of most interest, would be the change that results from the pain-relieving method employed. The sum of these two would give results as found. The apparent net trend is in the direction that is to be expected from the clear relationship demonstrated earlier between perceptual reduction and greater pain tolerance.

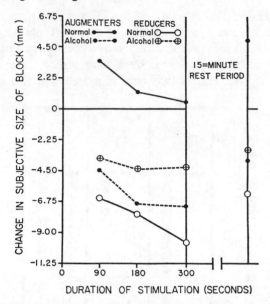

Fig. 15. Alcohol and normal: Effect of stimulation with large block for each group.

TABLE 5

Difference Between Alcohol and Neutral Sessions in Average Effect of Stimulation with Large Block

	Difference in Change in Estimated Size of Block (mm)				
	Duration of Stimulation (sec)			After 15-min rest	Standard Error of Difference Between Means
	90	180	300		
Augmenters ($N = 7$)	−7.92	−8.16	−7.56	−3.78	1.332
Moderates ($N = 10$)	1.92	0.81	0.96	1.11	0.963
Reducers ($N = 10$)	2.91	3.33	3.43	3.18	0.921

contributes to the manner in which this drug alleviates suffering with pain.

Alcohol and Reduction in Other Modalities

A diminution in the subjectively perceived intensity of sensation not only affects the intensity of sensations associated with pain but also those associated with discomfort and fatigue. When alcohol was consumed, the endurance of physical discomfort was increased in these subjects, as measured by the length of time each could hold his leg in an unsupported position. The well-known helpful effect of alcohol in seeming to provide a new lease of energy and comfort at times of fatigue may, indeed, partially be due to reduction in the perception of the symptoms of fatigue.

In spite of this diminished perception the consumption of alcohol is likely to interfere with effectiveness in sports where precision of movement is involved. The trained boxer, for example, who had taken alcohol, would be perceptually deceived about his own activities as well as those of his opponent. It is not surprising, therefore, that the consumption of alcohol during training is forbidden. (The street bully, on the other hand, may do better with a few drinks, insofar as his activity depends on the release of aggressive impulses; the trained boxer is attempting an act of skill.)

Not only does the reduction influence perceived size, weight, and pain, but the loudness of a sound of constant intensity is likely to be lessened after taking alcohol. The natural tendency when the loudness of one's own speech is diminished is for one to raise his voice. (This tendency can be observed in any beauty parlor, for when the client is under a hair dryer the noise of the machine masks her perception of the loudness of her own voice so that occasionally others overhear her telling her favorite manicurist what is clearly intended to be private.) At a cocktail party, if one is abstaining from drinking alcohol, the increasing loudness of the voices of the company is distinctly noticeable. When, however, one joins the drinking, the increase in sound passes unnoticed.

It is clear from the increased reduction following upon the intake of alcohol that the drug would make an augmenter more tolerant of pain and less tolerant of confinement. Thus one might predict that alcohol would encourage people to break out of confinement—out of a prison or a hospital—because it would decrease their tolerance for this situation, or for any situation that involves a diminution of changing sensory input. Such effects would be particularly pronounced in persons who, prior to taking alcohol, were at the augmenting end of the reactance continuum. Some evidence for this view is provided by the behavior of patients at the Boston Sanatorium. For example, when a patient leaves the sanatorium in the middle of treatment it is very frequently found that he has been drinking. Such self-discharges after drinking alcohol, moreover, occur most often in the type of patient who we know now is at the augmenting end of the reactance spectrum.

Similarities between the Effect of Alcohol and Prefrontal Lobotomy

The similarities between the effect of alcohol and of lobotomy have been frequently noted. In addition to the increased tolerance of pain, the greater carelessness of speech, lack of tact, and lower standards of social behavior of patients after lobotomy (Petrie 1952) are paralleled in some persons after the consumption of alcohol. A similarity between the effects of alcohol and of a lobotomy is found in other traits also. After taking alcohol the augmenter's perception of time has changed and his speed of performance has increased, while his self-criticism and his tendency to blame himself for failures have decreased. Moreover, after either alcohol or a lobotomy, the augmenter's endurance of discomfort is increased (Petrie 1952).

It is possible that the people examined before and after a prefrontal lobotomy in studies done in Europe (Petrie 1952 and 1958) tended to be augmenters and that the results of the lobotomy were colored because of this selectivity. This hypothesis is supported by the fact that the patients with intractable pain who sought this operation would, with certain exceptions, be likely to be the least tolerant of pain—that is to say, they would be augmenters. In addition, better results were reported for prefrontal lobotomy with neurotic patients suffering from anxiety and depression and both of these tendencies are characteristic of the introvert. Moreover, the few failures in the treatment of intractable pain by lobotomy were those with the personality type of the extravert (Petrie 1958). The positive relationship between extraversion and reduction and introversion and augmentation was discussed in chapter 2.

"Feigned Alcohol"

If alcohol alters perceptual reactance, then in every person whose life history includes the consumption of alcohol, the association between the drug and this alteration has been experienced. Pavlov's dogs, who normally experienced increased salivation with the intake of food, were soon found to salivate in response to cues that preceded the intake of food. It seemed probable that a consistent association of alcohol with an altered tendency to reduce might link this alteration with the cues that are associated with its consumption—that is to say, if we could reproduce these cues, we should be able to mimic the effect of alcohol. That is what we tried to do with what we have called "feigned alcohol" on the occasion, described above, when the liquid, in spite of all suggestions to the contrary, was non-intoxicating.

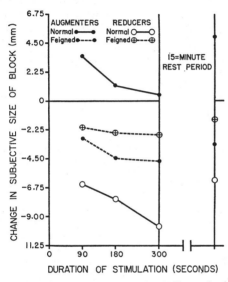

Fig. 16. Normal and "feigned alcohol": Effect of stimulation with large block for each group.

While the overall effect of real alcohol appears to increase the tendency for the group as a whole to reduce, that of "feigned alcohol" seems to decrease the tendency to reduce; but, when broken down, the results show that the augmenter augments less as a result of having had the "feigned alcohol" although the change is not as pronounced as it would be if he had had real alcohol. The reducers tend to reduce less, and the moderates remain pretty much unaltered (see Fig. 16). The changes in each perceptual subgroup with "feigned alcohol" thus parallel those found with real alcohol, although the relative weights of these changes are different. These findings support the hypothesis that the alteration in perceptual reactance induced by alcohol—or a similar drug—can be associated with cues that precede the consumption of alcohol.

If our interpretation of the effects of "feigned alcohol" as being a form of conditioning is correct for the perceptual subgroups, great care needs to be taken in any attempt to assess the efficacy of a commonly used drug by contrasting it with the effects of a "placebo." I suggest that the placebo would achieve a similar effect over a period of time as did the drug, and would be particularly effective for those people who are most susceptible to the drug. There may be a real possibility of helping such persons to gain indirect control of changes in perceptual reactance by using their associations with a drug that is effective in this area of involuntary behavior. In any event, it would be a great mistake to judge a drug as ineffectual because one seems able to achieve these results by the "suggestion" of a placebo.

ASPIRIN

Aspirin is one of the most useful drugs in the repertoire of the physician for the relief of pain and discomfort, but the manner in which it relieves such suffering is still a mystery. It may be that part of the effect of aspirin lies in its causing an increase, in some persons, in the tendency to reduce.

This drug, in contrast to alcohol and in the small doses in which it is commonly administered, has few recognized behavioral side effects and is not addicting. In a pilot study with hospital staff members, we have found that a mere two tablets of aspirin increase reduction. The most pronounced effect of this sort is on the augmenters who are changed so that they come to resemble the reducers.

Perceptual Reactance and Aspirin

The plan of the investigation followed exactly that used in the alcohol study. The 22 subjects were members of the staff of the Boston Sanatorium who had not been used in any previous study. Eleven of these subjects were augmenters, 9 were reducers, and 2 were moderates. Among the augmenters 3 were males, 8 females; among the reducers, 2 were males, 7 were females. The age range was from 32 to 67. Since the many duties of the hospital staff are likely to interfere with their return on the three occasions for the necessary period of time, maximum pressure was brought to bear on the reducers and augmenters to keep their appointments, for we required both for comparison. Thus, in this study, there is a pronounced shortage of moderates.

The routine dose was two tablets of aspirin, ground up, added to a glass of grapefruit juice, and drunk through a straw. First we

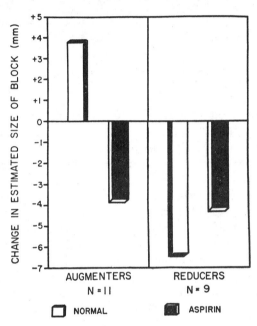

Fig. 17. Effect of aspirin.

obtained baseline scores on each subject with no drug. On the two subsequent occasions, either aspirin or "feigned aspirin" was administered in random order. A quantity of white harmless powder equal to two aspirins was ground up and added to the grapefruit juice in the session with aspirin "feigned." The experimenter and subject were told that this was an investigation of the effect of aspirin and aspirin-like drugs and were led to believe that active drugs were always contained in the grapefruit juice. The measurements of perceptual reactance were carried out half an hour after giving the aspirin.

The increased reduction of the augmenter with aspirin is highly significant (see Fig. 17 and Table 6). The scores of the reducers

TABLE 6

DIFFERENCE BETWEEN ASPIRIN AND NEUTRAL SESSIONS
IN AVERAGE EFFECT OF STIMULATION WITH LARGE BLOCK

	Difference in Change in Estimated Size of Block (mm)				
	Duration of Stimulation (sec)			After 15-min Rest	σ DM [a]
	90	180	300		
Augmenters ($N = 11$)	−7.41	−7.02	−8.55	−9.78	1.41
Moderates ($N = 2$)	0.93	−3.54	−5.73	−5.58	..
Reducers ($N = 9$)	1.32	2.40	2.88	0.33	1.86

[a] Standard error of difference between means under aspirin and neutral conditions.

and moderates, on the other hand, do not change significantly with aspirin. Nevertheless, when we take the usual approach to the estimation of a drug's effects—changes in the group as a whole—we find significantly increased reduction (.025 level of probability).

Some reduction occurs under conditions of "feigned aspirin," but it does not reach the level of significance. As there were many augmenters in this particular group, the effect of the "feigned aspirin" on the group as a whole was, as with alcohol, likely to be due largely to their susceptibility to the cues we provided.

Since the consumption of as little as two tablets of aspirin is followed by a significant increase in reduction, it is not unreasonable to suppose that this reduction contributes to the manner in which aspirin alleviates suffering with pain. This drug is likely to be most analgesic with the augmenter, to be less effective with the moderate and to cause little change in the reducer.

THE PRONOUNCED EFFECT ON AUGMENTERS OF PAIN-RELIEVING DRUGS

Alcohol and aspirin, both of which are associated with the increased tolerance of pain, produced a significant increase in reduction in augmenters. No augmenters continued to augment with either, but these drugs caused little or no significant change in reducers. Moreover, after a rest of a quarter of an hour the augmenters displayed significantly greater reduction for both drugs, while little or no change was noticeable in the reducers.

Not only do aspirin and alcohol have the maximum effect on augmenters, but within the group of augmenters we found the extreme augmenter more changed by the drug than the weak augmenter (see chapter 4).

Chlorpromazine

Earlier studies of the drug chlorpromazine indicated that it changes the personality toward the characteristics of the augmenter (Petrie 1958). Some isolated recent findings lend some further support to this view. For example, one of the stresses to which an augmenter is most vulnerable—bombardment with sound caused by the audioanalgesic apparatus (see next section)—was found to be intolerable to a patient given chlorpromazine on one of the days of testing. She said it was "too loud to bear." This patient, moreover, was the only one who retired completely from the experiment at a very early stage.

In addition, the one patient being treated with chlorpromazine included in the group of schizophrenic patients studied, was also the only patient found to augment on both of the occasions when he was tested. The other implications of these findings will be reported in the section on the schizophrenic.

The relationship between augmenting and the tolerance of confinement and restriction of activity is suggested in a report by S. Blough (1958) on the effect of chlorpromazine. He trained a bird to remain quietly on a particular spot for as long as five minutes. Then he gave the bird chlorpromazine and found that the amount of time the bird could remain still was substantially lengthened.

About Drugs in General

Although every observant physician notes the pronounced individual differences in the effect of drugs, experimental investigators have often tended to overlook such variation until relatively recently. Perhaps one cause of this oversight is that a large proportion of drug research is sponsored by drug companies. From the point of view of the manufacturers' sales the stress needs to be placed on the universality of the effects, rather than on their specificity. Moreover as we saw with the alcohol, a large minority of a sample population showing pronounced changes in one direction can significantly alter the picture for a whole group. It is of interest in this connection that if we were to examine a mixed group of people including augmenters, reducers, and moderates, a half hour after each had consumed two ounces of 80-proof liquor, we would discover that the temporary absence of augmenting behavior increases the homogeneity of the group; this might, in turn, contribute to the mistaken notions about the universal effects of the drug.

The form of behavior that results from changes in perceptual reactance, moreover, may be dependent on the environment in which these changes occur. An augmenter, having his alcohol with a group, may find he is increasingly tolerant of the group and its behavior. The same person, consuming his alcohol in a solitary room (confined in a TB sanatorium, say), may find his environment increasingly intolerable and, indeed, may leave the hospital and break off treatment as a result. Not only does the particular perceptual reactance determine the alteration caused by the drug, but also the particular environment in which that person finds himself determines his subsequent behavior. The conditions under which a drug is administered have been, perhaps, too often neglected.

The physiologist Michael Foster suggested one hundred years ago that what we need to know is how "sensation is fanned into the flame of pain." Further work in the areas outlined may contribute to our understanding of how the flame of pain—or another form of stress—may be subdued into acceptable sensation.

Perceptual Reactance Changed
4 by Sensory Stimulation

My external sensations are no less private to myself than are my thoughts or my feelings. F. H. BRADLEY (1846)

SENSORY STIMULATION CAUSING SUBDUED EXPERIENCE

We have discussed the decreased augmentation that follows upon the intake of alcohol and aspirin. Now we shall see that subdued sensation may be induced by changes in the external environment without the help of pain-relieving drugs.

When one considers the degree of augmentation that is shown under normal conditions at one end of the spectrum of perceptual reactance, it would seem that the augmenter ought to have some kind of built-in safety valve to protect him from being flooded when he is bombarded with sensation. Thus one may properly inquire whether augmenters possess any mechanism for subduing experience under conditions of heavy sensory bombardment. There is, indeed, some evidence in our work that the augmenter, when greatly stimulated, augments less. A hot bath is followed by decreased augmentation and exposure to extreme cold has similar results.

While I was preoccupied with these inquiries, I was undergoing dental treatment, and H. L. Ehrlich, a professor at the Harvard School of Dental Medicine, who has contributed at many levels to this research, agreed to substitute audioanalgesia for local anesthetic on two occasions when considerable pain was to be expected. Audioanalgesia is the recently developed method of attempting to increase tolerance for pain by exposing the patient at the time of his pain to stimulation with sound (Gardner, Licklider, and Weiss 1960). The intensity of the sound produced by this machine is under the control of the patient. When the treatment was in progress I turned the machine to its maximum setting and, in comparison with other occasions, was relatively free from pain. I noticed that when I experienced twinges of pain they were muted; they were more bearable to me than the accidental hurt that occurs usually in dental treatment.

Audioanalgesic methods have been experimentally used to increase the tolerance for pain of mothers during childbirth and of patients undergoing minor surgery, although the chief application, so far, has been in dental treatment. There is much controversy, partly because of the pronounced individual differences in its effects, as to the extent that audioanalgesia actually does increase tolerance for pain. If this method has such an effect, at once there arises the question of how it works. For example, in a recent report on audioanalgesia methods, Carlin and his associates say that "its successful use in the clinical situation depends both on distraction and suggestion" (Carlin, Ward, Gershon, and Ingraham 1962).

An Experiment with Audioanalgesia

An opportunity to explore systematically the effect of this kind of auditory stimulation upon kinesthetic reduction and augmentation was provided by the Harvard Dental School, where it was arranged for us to use their audioanalgesic apparatus on a group of outpatients.[1] The subjects were seen on two occasions and their perceptual reactance was measured by stimulation with the larger block. On one or the other of the occasions (the order was random), audioanalgesia accompanied the testing. The machine made by Bolt, Beranek, and Newman was used. Twenty-one subjects were drawn from among persons who had come to the Harvard School of Dental Medicine for treatment. When it became evident that it was going to be difficult for all of these patients to come on two occasions before their vacation, we asked the dental clinic to make a special effort to persuade those who clearly reduced or augmented without audioanalgesia to return for the second session, since the questions being asked concerned primarily the changes in the reducer and augmenter. The result of this differential persua-

[1] I am indebted to Dean Roy O. Greep and the staff of the Harvard School of Dental Medicine, and particularly to Harold L. Ehrlich, assistant clinical professor of dentistry at that school, who helped in many aspects of the research conducted there.

ion was that our population consisted of eleven augmenters, seven reducers and three moderates. (Might one, perhaps, find a dearth of reducers coming to a dental school for treatment since the reducer is more tolerant of the painful stimuli that urge others to seek treatment?)[2]

Each subject was first seen in a quiet room and occupied with some verbal tests for three-quarters of an hour while his hands were not used. The kinesthetic investigations for identifying the reducer and augmenter, as detailed in the appendix, were then carried out. The second session took place after an interval of at least 48 hours. On one or the other of these two occasions, the investigation was carried out while the patient was subjected to audioanalgesia, and this was arranged in random order.

When audioanalgesia was to be used, the subject was shown the machine and it was explained to him in some detail so as to minimize the strangeness of the procedure. In shape and size the apparatus is reminiscent of a mobile bedside table of the type used in hospitals. It needs to be connected with an electric outlet. Well-cushioned earphones for the patient's use are attached to the machine by a comfortably long lead. The experimenter also wore earphones, although these did not carry the sounds to which the patient was subjected, except during a brief period that was necessary for checking that all was in order.

In our experiment it was arranged that the patient heard "white noise" of moderate intensity through these earphones. White noise is the full acoustic spectrum of audible frequencies mixed together. (It sounds like "swish-sh" of intermediate pitch.) Stereophonic music can also be fed into these earphones.

The recommended method of treatment is first to let the patient hear only the stereophonic music that is played on tape and fed into the earphones for a few minutes and then to add the white noise. This procedure has the advantage of accustoming the subject to pleasant sound before the bombardment commences. It also enabled us to delay blindfolding the patient for the three minutes during which he listened to classical music.

As the patient is unable to hear any instructions once the earphones are in position, detailed instructions were given before the

[2] Sixteen of the subjects were female and five were male. Two of the augmenters, two of the reducers, and one of the moderates were male. The remainder in each subdivision were females. The ages ranged from 13 to 53.

music commenced. The patient's fingers were guided to the block in both cases, so that there was no appreciable difference in th methods used with and without the audioanalgesic apparatus.

Changes Following upon Stimulation with Sound

In every augmenter decreased augmentation was induced by stimulation with sound (see Table 7). The difference between th

TABLE 7

AUDITORY SENSORY STIMULATION AND PERCEPTION

| CATEGORIES | Subject | AVERAGE CHANGE IN ESTIMATED SIZE OF BLOCK IN MILLIMETERS | | |
		Score under Neutral Conditions	Score under Audiac	Difference
Augmenters	1	+13.59	−4.35	−17.94
	2	+7.44	−5.88	−13.32
	3	+6.96	−4.35	−11.31
	4	+4.14	+1.05	−3.09
	5	+5.13	−0.48	−5.61
	6	+3.48	−4.08	−7.56
	7	+2.01	−3.72	−5.73
	8	+1.71	−8.91	−10.62
	9	+0.96	−2.34	−3.30
	10	+0.27	−5.13	−5.40
	11	+0.24	−0.69	−0.93
Moderates	12	−2.61	−4.20	−1.59
	13	−2.79	−0.63	+2.16
	14	−3.90	+2.70	+6.60
Reducers	15	−3.12	−3.12	+0.00
	16	−5.16	−2.13	+3.03
	17	−5.37	−2.28	+3.09
	18	−6.69	−11.73	−5.04
	19	−6.99	−8.67	−1.68
	20	−7.80	−15.54	−7.74
	21	−8.70	+1.83	+10.53

average of their twelve scores with and without audioanalgesi (using a t test for differences between correlated means) wa significant at the .001 probability level (see Fig. 18).[3]

[3] Two augmenters were tested with small-block stimulation. Increase reduction with sensory bombardment was also observed with this procedure

No significant change was found in the reducers and moderates. The effect on the augmenters was, however, so pronounced that the data for the total mixed group of 21 show an increase in reduction that is significant at the .05-level of confidence. Nonparametric tests gave qualitatively the same conclusion. Moreover, after a quarter-of-an-hour rest the augmenters also displayed significantly greater reduction while no change was noticeable in the reducers.

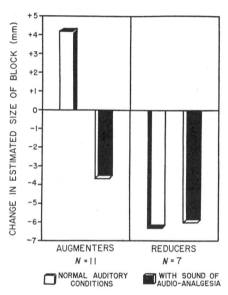

Fig. 18. Change with audioanalgesia.

The presumption is that under normal conditions we are measuring kinesthetically one aspect of the generalized tendency for the reducer to diminish his perception of all stimulation and for the augmenter to enlarge it. Let us infer for a moment that the auditory input supplied by the audioanalgesic apparatus is augmented by the augmenter, reduced by the reducer, and altered relatively little by the moderate. The prediction might then be made that the effect of auditory bombardment on these groups would bear out the manner in which they process the environment. In fact, in the spectrum from augmentation to reduction it is the augmenter who is the most affected by sensory bombardment; indeed, the greater his degree of augmentation, the more he is changed by the bombardment. The reducer remains almost unaffected and the moderate shows but slight changes that are in the same direction as the augmenter's. As we saw above, on the basis of a number of different approaches, a state of reduction is associated with higher tolerance for pain. Clearly auditory bombardment makes the augmenter reduce. Audioanalgesia might, therefore, be expected not to be universally effective; at any rate it is likely to be more useful to an augmenter.

Another limitation to the practical usefulness of relieving pain by accompanying white noise arises from the limited amount of time that one can safely subject a patient to this volume of sound. The recommended dose at present is no more than ten minutes at maximal strength, unless interrupted. In our research we kept the volume down to one-third of its maximum strength and limited the amount of time to eight minutes. One would suppose that during childbirth, for example, there would be already sufficient sensory bombardment to prevent hypoalgesia by the addition of white noise from being desirable or effective.

Dentistry is, of course, particularly suited to the use of audioanalgesia because the dentist keeps changing his tools and interrupts his treatment so that the pain is not continuous and the noise from the apparatus can be shut off intermittently. The ears then recover from the bombardment and can tolerate a further assault when the treatment begins once more.

It is nevertheless necessary to bear in mind that the sensitivity of the augmenter to sensory bombardment is manifested in his general reactions in addition to this increased reduction. For example, some of these patients said they would prefer dental pain to noise. The fact that the degree of reduction increases consistently after each period of stimulation—it is greater after 180 seconds than it is after 90 seconds, and still greater after 300 seconds—suggests that our figures may represent only a portion of the possible effect of prolonged sensory bombardment on the augmenter.

Bombardment with Other Sensations

The confirmation of our earlier finding that bombardment with sensation in one modality is followed by increased reduction in other modalities has many implications. For example, the effectiveness of the widely used treatment of pain by hot or cold packs— that is to say, by bombardment with thermal sensations—may be partly due to this mechanism. The fact that a patient, when in pain, appears to augment less than when he is free from pain suggests an explanation of an observation by Janet Travell (1959). She noted that patients do not complain of pain if an injection of novacaine is made while an area is painful; yet many complaints were made if such an injection was given in an area that was no longer painful. Nevertheless, it is not correct to identify the effect of bombardment by white noise in audioanalgesia with the effect of bombardment by sensory pain, for the former is steady and continuous, whereas pain is nearly always varying and modulated according to the stimulus conditions.

The increased reduction following upon bombardment with sensation is at least in part the explanation of the effectiveness of the counterirritant. For whether it is a medicine man using the greater pain of a burn to "drown the toothache" of his patient, or a nurse in our most modern hospital pinching the area of the patient's skin in which she is to give a hypodermic injection, each is accompanied by less augmentation.

Natural Reduction and "Defensive Reduction"

The reducer and augmenter appear to represent two ways of coping with stimulation when the intensity of such stimulation is not tailored to the individual needs of each. The reducer begins right away to limit the amount of stimulation impinging on him; the augmenter lays himself wide open to it and increasingly so. But we have seen that intense stimulation will, in the augmenter, produce temporary defensive reduction, so that the effect of such stimulation, to a certain extent, is self-limiting.

Pronounced, unsought stimulation, such as that from the volume of noise to which we are subjected, is increasing in our environment. We should note that at the augmenting end of the spectrum a person's usual perceptual reactance and his associated sensibilities and skills are the most threatened by such stimulation.

Comparison of Reduction Induced by Sensory Bombardment with That Produced by Drugs

Bearing in mind the possible attenuation of the change after sensory bombardment, it is nevertheless interesting to compare the effect on reduction of eight minutes of auditory stimulation with that following the ingestion of alcohol or aspirin. There is considerable agreement among these three procedures in the three groups of augmenters who have been the subjects of these separate studies in that augmentation is decreased by an average of 7.88 mm with alcohol, 7.65 mm with aspirin, and 7.71 mm with auditory sensory stimulation. (The numbers of augmenters were 7, 11, and 11 respectively.) The relative equality of the average change achieved by all three methods suggests that it may represent the average range of alteration in perceptual reactance that the augmenter possesses.

This change in perceptual modulation represents about one-quarter of the size of the measuring block. The difference in perceptual modulation between the extreme reducers and extreme augmenters, described in chapter 2, approximately equals the size of the measuring block. Therefore, the average change we have been able to induce is about one-quarter of the range between the extreme reducer and the extreme augmenter.

It is to be presumed that the degree of augmentation is also relevant to the effectiveness of these methods. A comparison of the extreme with the weak augmenters showed that after each of these three procedures decreased augmentation is most discernible for the extreme augmenters.[4] Indeed, a combination of the three groups showed that the change in the eleven extreme augmenters is significantly greater than in the remaining nineteen (at the .005 level of probability). The decreased augmentation of the extreme augmenters averaged 10.89 mm while that of the weak augmenters averaged 5.88 mm. The standard error of the difference between the means was 1.47.

Some Clinical Practices in Relation to Stimulation Causing Subdued Experience

In physical medicine, treatment of pain in muscle and joint is helped by moderate exercise of these areas.[5] Proprioceptive and other sensations coming in from our own bodies can contribute to

[4] Extreme augmenters are those who augment more than +3.00 mm on the large-block test under neutral conditions. Weak augmenters are those who augment less than +3.00 mm on the large-block test under neutral conditions. (On the small-block test a weak augmenter is designated as one who augments less than 6.00 mm under neutral conditions.)

[5] It appears that the explanation of greater pain tolerance based on increased circulation is no longer valid; nor has an alternative explanation been forthcoming (Schreiber 1962).

the tendency to reduction, so that the effectiveness of moderate exercise of the painful area may be partially due to the increased amount of such sensation engendered as a result of the exercise.[6] It may even be that the resultant reduction is partly why vigorous exercise has a certain quality of intoxication about it.

Bearing this in mind, let us consider the training in natural childbirth associated with the name of Grantly Dick Reed, or, for that matter, in painless childbirth, which is the term used by the Russians. It would seem—both from personal experience and the reports of investigators, such as that of Chertok (1959) in Paris —that such training is, in part, compounded as follows. The mother adds to the kinesthetic and visceral sensations coming to her from her own body others from the physical activities in which she has been instructed, thus decreasing her augmentation. She is taught to attend to these sensations, and to her physician and instructor, thus building up an association between such attention and decreased augmentation. We find with drugs how potent such an association can be in achieving decreased augmentation, and such association, we may infer, helps the mother also. Pain thus tends to become just one of many items in the totality of her sensations. In addition, she is told how to relax and thus to wait for the reduction that will set in as a result of the pain and all the other sensations associated with the birth of a child.

The augmenter, as we saw above, is quite properly the most apprehensive of pain. The training for natural childbirth breaks into the characteristic apprehensiveness of the augmenter with the explanations and reassurance it provides, as well as with the physical activity just discussed. Even if the aspects outlined are only partially contributory to the results obtained with natural childbirth, it is to be expected that the method will be most successful with certain patients, because of the characteristic effects produced on the augmenter by the various ways of increasing tolerance for pain.

Helping the Augmenter To Decrease His Vulnerability

Much of what has been said about childbirth, especially the fact that reduction follows upon bombardment with sensation including

[6] Phantom limb pain is an interesting example because when the amputee moves his body and limbs his pain is diminished.

pain, bears on how the augmenter can be helped to decrease his vulnerability. When the going is very tough he needs to attempt to wait in patience for the "second wind," that is, the reduction that will set in as a result of pain, and to try to concentrate on sensations other than pain while he is doing so.

Although distressing to the onlooker, crying may help to diminish suffering with pain because of the additional sensation it provides. The same advantages are associated with the characteristic rhythmic rocking and other movements performed by the person in pain. Nevertheless, the fact that we find exhaustion accompanying the reduction that follows upon extreme bombardment, needs to be borne in mind in deciding the extent to which such activity is encouraged.

The training of the augmenter should also, of course, make use of the findings on the favorable prospect of conditioning perceptual modulation. The fact that, for example, a glass of grapefruit juice that the subject thinks contains alcohol can achieve results that are an echo of those that occur with the alcohol present, gives some promise, also, for auto-conditioning. A patient could possibly make links for himself to the conditions that increase reduction— such as the feel and look of the bottle containing the aspirin—and then use those links to gain at least some remote control of the mechanism of reduction.

The possibility of gaining remote control of the mechanism of perceptual reactance is relevant also to assisting the reducer to increase his tolerance for the stresses to which he is most vulnerable. Such stresses are discussed in some detail in the chapter that follows.

THE PERCEPTUAL REACTANCE OF THE SCHIZOPHRENIC

It now seems fairly clear that auditory bombardment causes the augmenter to reduce defensively. Reduction also follows upon thermal bombardment. An augmenter, it might be predicted, is likely to reduce defensively in any environment that confronts him with more bombardment than he can tolerate. We have also seen that reduction in an augmenter can be triggered by a cue that has become associated with the potent stimulus for such a change. The greater the degree of augmentation under natural conditions, the more pronounced is such defensive reduction under conditions of overstimulation. Indeed, the greater the natural augmentation of the sensory bombardment, the more drastic does the defensive reduction need to be.

Schizophrenia is, of course, a multifaceted, very complex set of conditions with end product phenomena that seem to link them together. Nevertheless, the findings in a pilot study of seventeen schizophrenic patients become relevant here.[7] The schizophrenic's extraordinary tolerance of pain was the signal that led me to search for an association between reduction and the illness. For example, during this illness a lighted cigarette may be retained in the hand when it is burning the fingers, and severe self-mutilation may be practiced.

Apart from this kind of bizarre event that attracts attention to this insensitivity to pain, there exist such statistically tidy contrasts as appear between the number of dysmenorrhea sufferers among the staff of a mental hospital and the complete absence of dysmenorrhea among schizophrenic patients. But my own limited observations, combined with the wealth of those accumulated by gifted and careful physicians on these patients, suggested that their insensitivity during the schizophrenic phase of their illness contrasted with their sensitivity prior to its occurrence. One psychiatrist with great experience of these patients observed, "Where the schizophrenic lives there is much more intake than for the rest of us, so that they become abnormally sensitive to inflow" (Brill 1961).

As a heuristic hypothesis it appeared worth considering the possibility that the schizophrenic phase of the illness in some patients is accompanied by chronic and persistent reducing that is related to the "defensive reduction" following upon sensory bombardment. The results of the investigation of the perceptual reactance of these patients suggest that, although during the schizophrenic phase the great majority (82 per cent) were reducing, a considerable number (35 per cent) were shifting from extreme augmentation to extreme reduction, or vice versa, between the two occasions on which they were examined.

[7] The term "schizophrenic" is used in this volume to denote a person in the midst of episodes of active psychotic disorganization.

Seventeen schizophrenic patients at Toronto Psychiatric Hospital,[8] judged as representative by J. Lovatt Doust, were examined using stimulation with a larger block (a 1.5-inch block for measurement; a 2.5-inch block for stimulation). After an interval of at least one day, a second investigation was carried out on these same patients, using stimulation with a larger block of a different size (1 inch for measurement; 2 inch for stimulation). Because we have no other data on this particular combination of block sizes, it is necessary to report on reducing trends in terms of the proportion of the block reduced.

The Perceptual Stimulus-Barrier in Schizophrenia

Some of the findings are presented in Table 8 and the reader's attention is drawn to five points. The first is that all the schizo-

TABLE 8

PERCEPTUAL CHARACTERISTICS OF SCHIZOPHRENICS

| PERCEIVED CHANGE IN SIZE OF BLOCK | LARGE-BLOCK STIMULATION | | | |
| | First Occasion | | Second Occasion | |
	No.	Per cent	No.	Per cent
Reduced by one-sixth or more	13	77	12	71
Reduced by just less than one-sixth	1	6	2	12
Augumented by one-sixth or more	3	18	3	18
Total	17	100	17	100

phrenics but six reduced on both occasions; and most of them reduced to the extent of one-sixth or more of the measured block. This means that there were at least twice as many reducers among these schizophrenics as there were in any normal group we have studied (see Table 9).

[8] The Toronto Psychiatric Hospital arranged to send a psychologist to Boston for training in these methods and then made available to us the data on the patients with schizophrenia for statistical analysis and evaluation in comparison with the results of our previous studies and for subsequent communication. We are deeply appreciative of the cooperation of the hospital in this research, particularly to J. Lovatt Doust, the psychiatrist who stimulated my interest in applying concepts of augmentation and reduction to the study of schizophrenia, and also to I. Podniek, the psychologist who carried out the testing.

The second point is the sparcity of both moderates and augmenters among the schizophrenics.

Table 8 shows that the proportions of reducers and augmenters were practically identical on the two occasions but the table does not tell us the whole story, for the third point is that all of the patients reduced during one of the two testing sessions. That is to say, by the time of the second investigation, that tiny minority who had been augmenting had commenced to reduce and were replaced by three patients who had formerly reduced.

The fourth point is that the six patients who were reducing in one investigation and augmenting in the other were showing ex-

TABLE 9

PER CENT REDUCING BLOCK BY ONE-SIXTH OR MORE IN
SCHIZOPHRENIC GROUP COMPARED WITH OTHER GROUPS

Name of Group	Per cent Who Reduce Block by One-Sixth or More
Schizophrenics (on first occasion)	77 per cent ($N = 17$)
Schizophrenics (on second occasion)	71 per cent ($N = 17$)
Normal adults	35 per cent ($N = 23$)
Nurses	18 per cent ($N = 34$)

treme reduction and augmentation in comparison with all other groups studied. The increased oscillation of response in these schizophrenics is very large when the first test is compared with the second (see Table 10).

The degree of augmentation in four groups of normal augmenters was compared with that in the schizophrenics at each of the points in time when they were studied (90 secs, 180 secs, and 300 secs). On each occasion the schizophrenic augmenters were augmenting more than the four normal groups (see Table 11). The extreme degree of augmentation in the augmenting patients is another significant difference between the schizophrenics and the normals.

One patient is not included in this analysis because he had been given chlorpromazine before the two occasions on which he was tested. This man is the only schizophrenic in whom there was consistent augmenting behavior on *both* the occasions on which he

TABLE 10

CHANGE IN SCORES OF SCHIZOPHRENICS WHO REDUCED ON
ONE OCCASION AND AUGMENTED ON THE OTHER

	Subject	Score on First Occasion (mm)	Score on Second Occasion (mm)	Difference
Schizophrenics who reduced on the first occasion and augmented on the second occasion	1	−2.61	+3.24	5.85
	2	−5.58	+0.15	5.73
	3	−11.37	+8.88	20.25
Schizophrenics who reduced on the second occasion and augmented on the first occasion	4	+7.65	−2.07	9.72
	5	+11.61	−7.68	19.29
	6	+4.80	−5.43	10.23

was seen. That chlorpromazine changes patients in the direction of augmentation was suggested above and also in some earlier research (Petrie 1958).

So we come to the fifth finding about these schizophrenics—the persistence of the reduction once it had been induced. Thirty non-schizophrenics who reduced the size of the block by one-sixth or more were then compared with the ten schizophrenics who reduced to this extent on both testing sessions. After the 15-minute rest, the non-schizophrenic reducers were more than

TABLE 11

DIFFERENCE BETWEEN SCHIZOPHRENIC AUGMENTERS AND NORMAL AUGMENTERS

	CHANGE IN ESTIMATED SIZE OF BLOCK (MM)		
	Duration of Stimulation (sec)		
	90	180	300
Schizophrenics (N = 6)	+8.01	+6.08	+3.99
Group I—normal adults (N = 10)	+2.31	+0.39	+1.02
Group II—normal adults (N = 10)	+3.18	+3.60	+3.45
Group III—normal adults plus adolescents (N = 23)	+0.99	+0.67	+2.20

halfway back to their baseline, for their tendency to reduce was wearing off. It was not so with the schizophrenics, who were going down "deeper" than ever (see Fig. 19). The difference is significant at the .02 level of probability. On the second testing

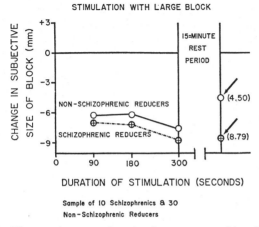

Fig. 19. The persistence of reduction among schizophrenic and non-schizophrenic reducers.

(the data of which do not appear in Fig. 19), the persistence of the reduction in schizophrenics was also apparent in that the degree of reducing was unchanged after the quarter of an hour of rest that followed upon the stimulation.

As the tendency to reduction wears off so much more slowly in the schizophrenics than in the others tested, it is not to be expected that the three-quarters of an hour hand-resting, routinely required prior to testing, would be as adequate a preparation for the schizophrenics as it is with other groups. Indeed, there is some suggestive evidence that the schizophrenics were in a state of reducing even after the three-quarter of an hour rest prior to the first set of measurements (see Appendix D). Suppose that we had retested the normal group, shown in Figure 19, after the quarter of an hour rest that followed the testing, when they were still reducing by 4.50 mm. Whatever scores we then obtained would have been an underestimation of their reduction by at least 4.50 mm. This merely means that the degree of reduction in the schizophrenics depicted on this graph is presumably an *underestimation* of their real tendencies.

Some Reflections on the Perceptual Reactance of Schizophrenics

What is clearly apparent in the schizophrenic group is that in the majority of these patients there is a restriction on intake from the environment during their state of illness. It might, with further research, be possible to spell out how this stimulus-barrier in perception results from the interaction of the particular nervous system the schizophrenic inherited with the environment to which he is subsequently subjected. It will be recalled that the way in which sensory bombardment causes subdued experience suggests how reduction may be induced in nonschizophrenic augmenters by special conditions in the environment. Further work with this approach might throw light on the preponderance of a somewhat special type of reduction in the schizophrenic. For the present, we must content ourselves with noting that the schizophrenic's extreme tolerance of pain during his illness fits with his special perceptual reactance. (Indeed, some workers regard increased sensitivity to pain in a schizophrenic as an indication that the patient is improving.) The lack of differentiation between stimulation from outside and inside himself may also be due to the attenuation of these sensations as a result of reduction.

It will be noted in the next section that among those who were born deaf, but not among those who became deaf later in life, there were fewer reducers than in the normal group. One wonders whether the very early occurrence of this adaptive alteration, in their case in the direction of augmentation, also provides a clue as to the timing of an adaptive alteration in the direction of reduction—one that occurs in the presence of over-stimulation. Might it be that the withdrawal of the schizophrenic into a special type of reduction was also learned very early in development?

When the schizophrenic goes into what may be called his spasm of reduction, it is not a carefully modulated procedure in which he reduces just enough for his convenience. Rather, he is seemingly forced by his own sensibility to go to an extreme. In this extreme state of reduction the world may become unbearable—not because of what it contains, but because of what it does *not* contain. The schizophrenic finds himself having to cope with a new problem— the problem of being confronted with nothingness. The psychotic experiences that then occur might be thought of as creating a world in which the schizophrenic can live. The function of hallucinations in increasing sensory input during periods of sensory lack was discussed earlier in connection with experimental confinement and isolation (chapter 2).

The hallucinatory experiences may have enhanced value for the schizophrenic during his illness because they provide fresh stimulation. Reduction, it will be remembered, is a process occurring in time. In the schizophrenic, once reduction is induced, it is significantly more persistent than in the normal group. Fresh stimulation has the advantage of not yet having been subjected to the spasm of reduction that is characteristic of the schizophrenic.

It is tempting to speculate further as to how prophylaxis and treatment might be better adapted to the perceptual characteristics and associated vulnerabilities of the schizophrenic. For example, if a patient is in the process of coming out of his schizophrenic state, it may be important to protect him from too much stimulation, so that his defensive reduction will not be reactivated.

In any event, the findings reported lend support to the heuristic hypothesis that some schizophrenics were originally augmenters— indeed the more pronounced type of augmenters—who were confronted with more bombardment than they could tolerate, internal as well as external. During their illness, they are subjected to what might be called spasms of defensive reduction, but there are phases, even then, when they return temporarily to their natural, augmenting selves. Such a reconstruction finds support among the historians of schizophrenia, who describe these patients as originally being persons of exquisite sensibility, indeed, as showing pathological hyperesthesia.

The Impact of the Lack of One Sense Modality on Perception

Bombardment with sound causes the augmenter to reduce but has no significant effect on the reducer. It seemed reasonable to suppose that the effect on perceptual style of lack of stimulation—for example, lack of auditory stimulation in those persons born deaf—would be the reverse of that of its overstimulation. The effect would be noticeable at the reducing end of the reactance spectrum and would consist of diminished reduction.

Moreover, it would seem likely that the amount of alteration following upon the chronic lack of auditory stimulation would be less than that following upon temporary traumatic bombardment with auditory sensation. Hence one would expect to find in a population that was born deaf a dearth of extreme reducers. These effects of auditory lack might also be present, although to a lesser extent, in persons who became deaf during the course of their lives.

A STUDY OF THE DEAF

A study of the perceptual reactance of the deaf population of Nashville, Tennessee, was carried out under the direction of Shalom E. Vineberg, by Miss G. Kratz. Their results on 27 deaf people, of whom 12 had been born deaf and 15 had become deaf at some time after birth, were compared with a population of 45 of like age and similar occupation with normal hearing. Large-block stimulation was used.[9] The proportion of persons reducing the size of the block by an average of 5.4 mm was 0 per cent in those born deaf and 29 per cent in those with normal hearing, and this difference is highly significant. Those who became deaf after birth do not differ significantly from those with normal hearing.[10]

Some Reflections on the Perceptual Reactance of the Deaf

The finding that in those born deaf there is a dearth of reducers suggests that adaptation occurs to a lack of stimulation as well as to excess of stimulation. The implication of this finding is that deaf persons are able to obtain, through all modalities other than hearing, some extra information and stimulation that may be an important factor in their successful adaptation to their birth defect.[11] The fact that significant differences are found in those who were born deaf in contrast to those who became deaf points to the possibility

[9] I am greatly indebted to Shalom E. Vineberg, professor of psychology at the University of Houston, and Miss G. Kratz for the time and effort devoted to this study.

[10] In both deaf groups no relationship was found between the amount of reduction and the sex or I.Q. of the subject.

[11] Many of the deaf examined were printers. Greater manual dexterity and accurate performance at the augmenting end of the spectrum is to be expected (Petrie 1952).

that perceptual adaptation to a sensory lack is most successfully achieved in early youth.

Lack of auditory sensation may, however, have rather special effects. One obvious contrast between hearing and seeing is that when our senses are intact the auditory world is always with us; we can shut our eyes but not our ears. Moreover, the voice of the mother often provides the baby, even when he does not see her, with clues to the existence of a loving and safe environment, which he can otherwise understand only from the physical warmth and support that originally is the mother for him. It is not impossible that sounds, especially in contrast to sights, may continue to be loaded with special emotional significance. The special role played by sound in the stability of an individual is also suggested by the characteristic personality difficulties that occur in the deaf as compared with the blind. Thus we cannot regard the adaptation to loss of hearing as necessarily being representative of adaptation to any other sensory loss.

During the kinesthetic investigation of perceptual reactance the patient is blindfolded. (See instructions in Appendix.) One other point (of which Vineberg was well aware) is that when the eyes of a deaf person are covered, his sensory lack is temporarily still further increased. Part of the change toward the augmenting end of the spectrum may be due to such further deprivation. But even should this be the case, it would merely emphasize the potentialities for perceptual adaptation in those who are sensorially deprived. This type of adaptation is the obverse of that found in those who are sensorially overstimulated.

Indeed, however interesting the pathological examples may be, the main intent of this chapter was to show that in the vast "normal" population, perceptual reactance and vulnerability to different kinds of suffering can be changed by pronounced sensory stimulation.

The Perceptual Reactance of
5 Juvenile Delinquents and of
Alcoholics

The calm that cooles thine eye does shipwrack mine, for O,
Unmov'd to see one wretched is to make him so.

RICHARD CRAWSHAW (1649)

THE STIMULUS-GOVERNED

In the course of this research an additional but atypical perceptual
style emerged. The pattern was noted in the first instance in those
patients seen in the hospital, in whom there turned out later to be
clinical indications of brain pathology.[1] This perceptual type can be
designated as stimulus-governed. The stimulus-governed individual, as can be seen in Figures 20 and 21, is characterized by the
fact that when a larger object is used for stimulation, he reduces
the measured block by 6 mm or more (on the extreme set of
measurements among the three trials) and when stimulated with a
smaller object he increases it by more than 6 mm. It will be
remembered that the contrast effect of the smaller stimulus tends to
encourage augmenting and inhibit reducing, whereas that of the
larger stimulus encourages reducing and inhibits augmenting.
Hence these stimulus-governed persons can be thought of as displaying to an exaggerated degree the normal contrast effect of the
juxtaposed sizes; that is to say, such a person is least able to escape
from the direct and restrictive influence of the relative size of the
juxtaposed stimuli.

[1] I am indebted to James R. Gallacher, professor of pediatrics, for the
facilities made available to us at the adolescent clinic of the Children's
Medical Center of Harvard Medical School, and to H. A. Ravin, formerly
head of the department of neurology at Beth Israel Hospital, for his assistance.

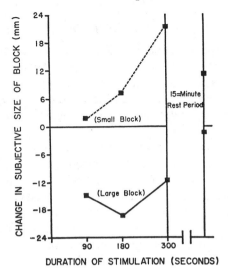

Fig. 20. L. E., male with clinical indications of brain pathology—stimulation with large and small blocks.

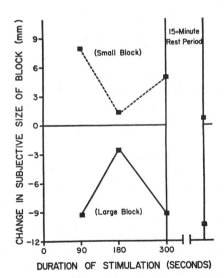

Fig. 21. L. M., female with diagnosis of occipital lobe disease—stimulation with large and small blocks.

A STUDY OF JUVENILE DELINQUENTS

The term juvenile delinquent covers a very heterogeneous population, whose behavior is diverse and complex. My own observations of some members of this heterogeneous group and the reports of those who know them well alerted me to the fact that delinquents in general are quite tolerant of pain and intolerant of the stress of confinement. Opinions vary as to whether these characteristics are merely a motivational affair of the personality or whether they have, in addition, some more fundamental physiological base. We have laid down the hypothesis that, in addition to having poor homes, a large number of juvenile delinquents have certain unrecognized perceptual needs and consequent vulnerabilities and that their education and treatment are not well adapted to relieve some of these needs. Moreover, the general conduct of certain delinquents is reminiscent of that of some brain-injured patients. For these reasons we proposed to explore the possible role of perceptual abnormality and sensory insufficiency in the development of delinquent behaviour.

The People Studied

Our study originally sampled some 70 delinquent girls and boys between the ages of thirteen and seventeen, in three institutions in Massachusetts where they were detained.

This particular group was limited to white, right-handed adolescents. (The additional variables to be taken into account with a left-handed person are discussed below.) Those with neurological conditions or known psychiatric problems, or those who had taken any kind of medicine or drug on the day of testing were excluded. As controls, girls and boys of like age-group were studied in the public schools ($N = 25$) and in a nurses' training school ($N = 37$), also in Massachusetts (see Figs. 22 and 23).

The number of reducers and augmenters and moderates turned out to be almost exactly the same among the boys and the girls in all the subgroups, so that sex differences have not contributed appreciably to the findings.

Perhaps of greater importance is the comparability in respect to reactance type of the group from the nurses' training school to the group from the public high school, for there is always the chance

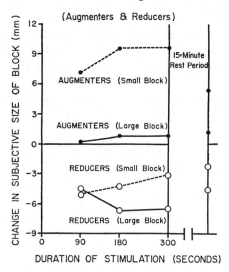

Fig. 22. The non-delinquent adolescents—stimulation with large and small blocks (Augmenters and reducers).

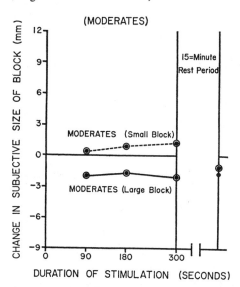

Fig. 23. The non-delinquent adolescents—stimulation with large and small blocks (Moderates).

that the sample of school children that chooses to devote the time necessary for two prolonged investigations is atypical of the group being studied. The nurses were, however, instructed to take part and had no option in the matter; thus we were sure in their case that we had an unbiased sample of the nursing school. The comparability of this group with that from the public school reassured us as to the representativeness of the latter.

The Proportion of Juvenile Delinquents Who are Stimulus-Governed

Fourteen of these delinquents showed the atypical stimulus-governed behavior, as against only three of the non-delinquents.

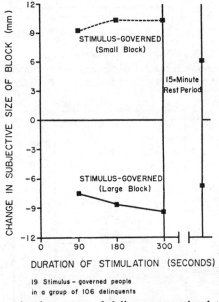

Fig. 24. The stimulus-governed delinquents—stimulation with large and small blocks.

The difference is significant below a P value of .01.[2]

Strong stimulus-governed behavior was defined as applying to a person who reduced the measured block by 5.4 mm or more on the average of 12 measurements when stimulated with a larger block

[2] Details are presented in Appendix B showing that stimulus-governed reactions to the perception of size are associated with atypical behavior in the perception of weight.

and who increased his estimate to the same extent when stimulated with a smaller block. With this criterion, 17 per cent of the delinquents were classed as strongly stimulus-governed, whereas no non-delinquent qualified. That difference is significant beyond a *P* value of .001. Moreover, in a study conducted in the past few months of another group of 36 male juvenile delinquents, 20 per cent were found to be strongly stimulus-governed while none quali-

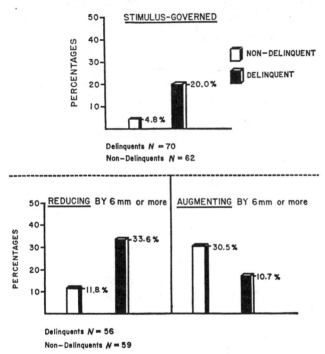

Fig. 25. Contrast in percentages showing three different perceptual styles in the delinquent and non-delinquent groups.

fied in a further group of 34 non-delinquents. (The *P* value is .01; see Fig. 24.) It will be recalled that the stimulus-governed pattern appeared in the first instance in patients in hospitals in whom there turned out to be clinical indications of brain pathology (compare Figs. 20 and 21 with Fig. 24). Thus a perceptual abnormality of a kind, one that might be said to signify a lack of "perceptual homeostasis," is a factor in approximately one out of every five juvenile delinquents studied, totaling now more than one hundred. (See Fig. 25.)

The Behavior of the Stimulus-Governed Delinquents

These stimulus-governed delinquents had committed more delinquencies than the others by the time they were investigated; 47 per cent of the stimulus-governed, as compared with 19 per cent of the remainder, had committed five or more delinquencies. (The numbers in the two groups were 17 and 64 respectively.) The difference is significant. Their delinquency had started somewhat earlier, but this difference was not significant.

Among the delinquencies for which these delinquents are officially recorded as having been detained, are the following: armed robbery, assault and battery, assault on a principal (presumably a school principal), attempted rape, possession of BB guns, breaking and entering, larceny of motor vehicle, driving without a license, drunkenness, larceny, stealing candy, trespassing, truancy, violation of probation, and window-breaking.

The juvenile delinquents were assessed by supervisors, who were in constant contact with them, and notes were made of their behavior and their history during the time that they were in the institution. It was from these notes and assessments that some further differences between the stimulus-governed delinquents and the remainder were elicited. The stimulus-governed were mentioned more frequently as being "immature, unpredictable, changeable." Forty-one per cent of the stimulus-governed were so designated as compared with 10 per cent of the remainder. (The numbers on whom assessments were available were 17 and 60 respectively.) These differences are highly significant.

It should be expected that the reactions of the stimulus-governed would be likely to appear unpredictable and unsuitable to an onlooker who is not experiencing the contraction and expansion of the sensory environment that appears to characterize their perceptions. The motivation of such a delinquent remains a mystery to the people around him, who perceive the world in a much more stable fashion than he does and whose vulnerabilities and strengths are consequently also more constant than are his.[3]

[3] The stimulus-governed delinquent does not have noticeably inferior intellectual equipment. He is broadly comparable in intelligence to the rest of the delinquent group in that his average Wechsler I.Q. is 96.6, while the average for the remainder is 98.0.

Stimulus-Governed Tendencies and Immaturity

Some abnormalities simply represent the absence of mature patterns. It may well be that the stimulus-governed perceptual style is normal in early infancy, for evidence is accumulating that stimulus-governed behavior is associated with what may be called extreme immaturity.

As reported earlier in this chapter, the strong stimulus-governed pattern did not appear in the control groups. It seemed desirable, however, to try to measure the tendency toward stimulus-governed behavior in different age-groups by examining the difference between the large-block and small-block scores—a difference that indicates the susceptibility to contrast effects. The amount of spread between these two averages was the measure used. The hypothesis explored was that there is a trend, as we approach childhood, for the spread to increase between the small-block and large-block scores.

The subjects included adolescents who ranged from 14 to 18 years, students from 18 to 26, and adults from 33 to 56 years. The results showed a progression in the susceptibility to these contrast effects from the adults to the students, and then from these to the adolescents (see Table 12).

TABLE 12

STIMULUS-GOVERNED TENDENCIES FOR
DIFFERENT AGE-GROUPS

Name of Group	Average Spread Score (mm)
Adolescents Age: 14–17	6.15 ($N = 25$)
Student Nurses Age: 18–26	5.49 ($N = 33$)
Adults Age: 33–56	4.74 ($N = 15$)

The Youngest Age Groups

The techniques of testing required that we limit the study to children mature enough to understand the instructions. An intelligent child of six, used to hearing precise verbal explanations in his own home, could comprehend the instructions but these six-year-olds were the lowest age-group that provided reliable results.

Studies of young children were carried out at Woods Hole, Massachusetts, and in Lincoln, Massachusetts.[4] For the purposes of the statistical analysis, the children were divided into two groups—those who were six or seven years old and those who were eight to twelve years old.

The size of the children's hands necessitated the use of smaller blocks than those described in the standard procedure.[5] In order to have comparable scores, all the measurements made with the different size of blocks were multiplied by a ratio of block sizes, thus keeping the ratios constant. This procedure was somewhat arbitrarily adopted in order to have a system of scores. The spread, as expressed by percentage of the block used, appears to increase as we pass from the group aged eight to twelve to that aged six or seven—from 16.61 per cent to 21.81 per cent. The adult spread is 12.44 per cent of the block.

What all this means is that there exists some evidence that, as maturity advances, the stimulus-governed type of behavior tends to decrease. The argument, of course, stems from the range of spread that we have been able to ascertain so far. It is possible that younger children might show the degree of spread found in the stimulus-governed adolescent.

It would seem that these turbulent stimulus-governed tendencies normally become more controlled and restrained as maturity increases. The delinquent stimulus-governed person, however, fails to develop this control and continues his life exposed to an unpredictably expanding and contracting sensory environment.

A Comparison of the Dominant and Non-Dominant Hand

There is another finding that suggests that with increasing experience one learns to restrain and control perceptual susceptibility to

[4] Situated at Woods Hole, Massachusetts, are both the Marine Biological Laboratory and the Woods Hole Oceanographic Institution. Included in this group are children of the scientists and technicians who had moved to this area because of these institutions, and also children of the local population. In Lincoln, Massachusetts, are many parents whose work takes them to the universities and industries in the adjacent areas.

[5] *Lincoln children*. The measuring block for large-block stimulation was ¾-inch and for small-block stimulation 2 inches. *Woods Hole children*. The measuring block for large-block stimulation was 1 inch and for small-block stimulation was 1½ inches.

contrast effects. It arises from the differences to be expected between the more accustomed hand and the hand that is less frequently used. If in normal maturation the tendency toward stimulus-governed behavior is increasingly controlled and restrained, then this control should be more pronounced in the dominant hand. I wondered whether the left hand in right-handed people and the right hand in left-handed people would not tend to show susceptibility to these contrast effects to a greater extent than does the customarily used hand.

In a small sample of twelve reducers, augmenters, and moderates, the findings indicated that there was significantly greater spread in the non-dominant hand. As will be seen in Table 13, the

TABLE 13

STIMULUS-GOVERNED TRENDS IN DOMINANT
AND NON-DOMINANT HANDS
(FOR RIGHT-HANDED SUBJECTS)

NAME OF GROUP	AVERAGE SPREAD SCORE (mm)	
	Dominant Hand	Non-Dominant Hand *
Reducers (N = 4)	7.29	10.89
Moderates (N = 6)	3.42	5.01
Augmenters (N = 2)	7.41	15.72

* The difference between the spread scores of the dominant hand and the spread scores of the non-dominant hand for the total group is significant at the .05 level for a two-tail test. The Wilcoxen Matched-Pairs Signed-Ranks test was used.

trend is toward a greater susceptibility to these contrast effects in the unaccustomed hand in all three reactance categories.

In a further small study of four left-handed moderates, it was also found that the spread is greatest in the non-dominant hand—in this case the right hand. Thus we found the control of stimulus-governed behavior trends more pronounced in the dominant hand in all the groups studied. These findings about the dominant hand support the hypothesis that in normal development, with increasing experience, one learns to control and restrain stimulus-governed behavior. The results also underscore the importance of ascertaining the handedness of a subject before measuring his perceptual reactance (see instructions in Appendix A).

Fatigue

Fatigue, it was thought, might lead to some regression in perceptual reactance, as it does in other areas of behavior. There does indeed seem to be an association between fatigue and the weakening of the control that restrains perceptual susceptibility to contrast effects. In a small group of subjects who were studied in the morning and afternoon, it was found that, as the day wore on, and fatigue increased, stimulus-governed trends also increased. The average spread between large-block and small-block scores, which had been 5.58 mm early in the day, became 7.41 mm later in the day in the six subjects studied in this manner. (The standard error of the difference between means is 2.49.)

The amount of change with fatigue noted in this group, moreover, is likely to be attenuated. The special circumstances of the institution where they were housed precluded our seeing these particular subjects very late in the day; there was, therefore, less time than we would have wished prior to the second investigation for pronounced fatigue to be manifested. It is clear, however, that one should not attempt to measure a person's characteristic perceptual reactance when the person is in a state of fatigue (see instructions in Appendix A).

Differentiating the Schizophrenic from the Stimulus-Governed Perceptual Reactance

The question needs to be raised whether it is possible that the schizophrenics discussed in chapter 4 (who were examined in two sessions, using two different sizes of large-block stimulation) might, with our later techniques, turn out to be similar to the stimulus-governed.

The most characteristic aspect of schizophrenic reduction, in comparison with normal reduction, is its prolonged nature (chapter 4). So we compared the stimulus-governed with the schizophrenic group with regard to this variable, and the persistence of reduction was found to be significantly greater in the schizophrenic than in the stimulus-governed group. We used the score after 15 minutes of rest in the large-block stimulation sessions. Thus, the most characteristic difference between schizophrenic and normal reduction holds up also in comparing the schizophrenics with the stimulus-governed.

In addition, Dr. Julian Silverman, of the National Institute of Mental Health, Bethesda, Maryland, subsequently carried out studies of schizophrenics using the perceptual reactance approach (Silverman 1964 and 1966). He confirms our finding that withdrawn, non-paranoid schizophrenics, who form the bulk of schizophrenics confined in mental hospitals, show a special form of reduction, and he includes other very interesting data. In his study both large- and small-block stimulation were used. His findings are therefore particularly valuable in further differentiating the schizophrenic from the stimulus-governed. Further studies of the schizophrenic with this differentiation in mind would be most valuable.[6]

It is, of course, not possible to identify the stimulus-governed when scores on only one size of block are available. Before finding this atypical form of perceptual modulation a number of such investigations were carried out. Fortunately, the other earlier findings mentioned previously, when we were still using stimulation with only one size of block, were based on work with adult subjects, and those with any history of neurological or psychiatric involvement had been excluded. As was explained above, we have found stimulus-governed reactions, among adults, only in the presence of neurological or psychiatric abnormality. Therefore, it is very unlikely that the samples studied included stimulus-governed persons.[7]

It is necessary, however, to complete sessions with both sizes of

[6] Such differentiation is particularly desirable in comparing the stimulus-governed reaction with the oscillation of response found in one-third of the schizophrenics included in the original study described in chapter 4.
Further data that has just become available from the Langley Porter Clinic in San Francisco makes it clear that stimulus-governed reactions are not characteristic of schizophrenics, although it appears in a small proportion of those studied. Enoch Calloway, psychiatrist at that clinic, will be continuing with some very fruitful research in this whole area.
[7] A sample of the subjects were examined with small-block stimulation in the investigation of the effects of sensory bombardment, and decreased augmentation was demonstrated. Thus we were reassured that stimulus-governed behavior was not being induced by this procedure. Moreover, a reexamination of the changes following upon administration of the pain-relieving drugs provided considerable evidence that the subjects had not become stimulus-governed after these approaches either.

blocks in order to identify this atypical form of perceptual modulation (see instructions in Appendix A).

False Stimulus-Governed Scores

A word of warning is proper here. It is occasionally possible to
obtain a false stimulus-governed score. If, for example, prior to the
testing with the large stimulus, the patient had been subjected to a
drug, or to one of the other means by which an augmenter can be
changed into a reducer, we would obtain an induced reducer score
yet, if he were tested without any such interference with the small
block, he would give us an augmenter score. The large number of
delinquent youngsters showing stimulus-governed behavior cannot,
however, be accounted for in any such manner.

Some Reflections on Stimulus-Governed Trends

To understand the seemingly volcanic characteristics of the stimulus-governed person, the ups and downs of his emotions, his occa-
sional over-reactivity, and his unpredictability, we need to remember his mercurial perceptual characteristics—the fact that he is
subjected to the direct and restrictive influence of the relative size
of the juxtaposed stimuli. For him the sensory environment would
seem to be contracting and expanding in size and in intensity,
depending upon external chance events.

It would appear that the turbulence of the stimulus-governed
trends, the extreme swings from expansion to contraction, in accordance with the contrast in the stimuli provided by the environment, are controlled and restrained as the normal individual ma-
tures. Thus, the perceptually mature individual, be he reducer,
augmenter, or moderate, is subjected to only a limited extent to the
pressures of such contrast effects.

There are many pointers associating stimulus-governed behavior
with immaturity. The good mother is warm and permissive about
the continual shifts in her young child's preoccupation and emotions. Similar warm and permissive behavior could be a source of
reassurance and comfort in the life of the adolescent who has the
misfortune to be stimulus-governed, although he, like the child,
may also need to have limits set. Refined educational techniques
will be required, as it seems that this particular type of immaturity

does not affect intelligence but is most likely to influence the affective life—to influence what motivates him and what attracts him. The fact that in other ways he can be compared with children of his own age will demand great understanding from the adults around him, on whom he may need to depend to take him in tow.

The Driving of Motor Cars by Adolescents

Not every adolescent who drives dangerously is to be labeled a juvenile delinquent, yet as we are fast approaching a condition in western countries where the loss of life due to disease is less than that due to traffic accidents, it is as well to look at any prophylactic hints about dangerous driving that can be found.

There is ample evidence that a disproportionate number of accidents are caused by adolescent drivers. Stimulus-governed trends are still present in the adolescent; this implies that precise perceptual adaptation may be made difficult for him by the subjective expansion and contraction of his sensory environment.

It might be well on both theoretical and practical grounds to carry out further research on the maturation of perceptual reactance. The findings might prove helpful in identifying a high-risk group and might also contribute to our knowledge of the lowest age at which driving permits could wisely be granted.

Some Theoretical and Neurological Points

Of course, what we do not know as yet is whether the stimulus-governed adolescent is likely to remain in this atypical state forever, or whether phases of maturation that would serve to stabilize his perceptual life are simply late in developing. Nor can we be sure that with eventual perceptual maturity, it may not be too late for him to change his self-concept and to lose the habits that he has accumulated and to alter the circumstances that he has arranged around himself during the sixteen years when he was being pushed first in one direction and then in the other by his perceptual environment.

A possibility that needs to be borne in mind is that the stimulus-governed found among juvenile delinquents and among the special patients in hospital who were examined may have this atypical pattern as a result of different causes. The stimulus-governed delinquent may be displaying extreme slowness of devel opment, and it is primarily his extreme immaturity that is respon sible for his condition. On the other hand, stimulus-governec behavior found in conjunction with serious brain pathology may be a form of regression from maturity due to acquired pathology

Some of the stimulus-governed persons show changes within the five minutes of stimulation (see Fig. 21). The possibility cannot be excluded as yet that stimulus-governed behavior is displayed inter mittently, as is frequently the case with neurological signs. These swings within the five minutes may, of course, also have their own place in the developmental sequence.

The method described here appears to be effective in detecting some atypical perceptual characteristics that have not been dis cerned with other techniques. For example, tracings showing the changes in electric potential produced by the brain in the waking drowsing, and sleeping phases have been obtained on seven delin quent stimulus-governed boys. Mary L. Scholl kindly arranged to provide written interpretations of their records at Beth Israel Hos pital in Boston. Electroencephalographic abnormality was discerni ble in only one of these boys and he did not show the more extreme stimulus-governed behavior. It would seem that atypicality asso ciated with the stimulus-governed is a characteristic not reflected in the electrical activity of the cortex as currently recorded and usually interpreted. (Of course, there are other forms of atypical ity, like mongolism, which are not obviously reflected in the usual electroencephalographic recordings.)

Our findings also indicate that the immaturity of perceptual reactance in the stimulus-governed person does not affect the ma turing of his intelligence. It may well be that, in normal develop ment, some special aspects of the nervous system inhibit these perceptual contrast effects.

Just as blindness can inform us only to a limited extent about the functions of the seeing eye, the alterations accompanying lesions in the brain can contribute only to a limited extent to our understand ing of the brain's function when it is intact. Nevertheless, the change in perceptual reactance that appears to be associated with lesions in the frontal areas suggests that somewhere in this large neural circuit may lie the control of perceptual reactance that develops during normal maturation (Petrie 1958).

It is of interest that lesions of different extent in the frontal regions—and in the thalamic nuclei with which they are connected —are not accompanied by electroencephalographic changes (Petrie 1952 and 1958). Nor, as we have seen, is immaturity of perceptual reactance associated with atypical electroencephalographic recordings.

Does Sensory Insufficiency Contribute to Delinquency?

The hypotheses that underlay the research [8] described in this chapter were that in addition to having poor homes, a large number of that heterogeneous group known as juvenile delinquents have certain perceptual needs and consequent vulnerabilities, and we had set out to explore the possible role of perceptual abormality and sensory insufficiency in the development of delinquent behavior. We have discussed the evidence for the existence of vulnerabilities due to perceptual abnormality in some juvenile delinquents; now let us turn to the problems associated with sensory insufficiency.

Two aspects of the delinquent's behavior contributed particularly to this part of the hypothesis. The delinquent is remarkably stoical with pain and he is intolerant of monotony and restriction of activity.

Since the reducer reverses the behavior of the augmenter in respect to both pain and sensory insufficiency (tolerating pain well but suffering when subjected to monotony, isolation, and restriction of activity), we undertook to explore the possible contributary role of sensory insufficiency in the development of delinquent behavior.

In the preceding section findings are detailed that make it necessary to consider the perceptual reactance of the stimulus-governed juvenile delinquents separately from the rest of the group. We have

[8] The research on delinquents reported in this section owes much to Mrs. Rook McCulloch who created the conditions for commencing these investigations, and to Mary L. Scholl, instructor in neurology at Harvard Medical School, who reported on the EEG investigations of a pilot group of delinquents. Francis Kelly of the Division of Youth Service of the Commonwealth of Massachusetts and the staff at the Reception Center for Boys in Roslindale have been exceedingly cooperative about this research. Jacob Schonfield now professor at the University of Maryland Medical School made all the arrangements for the investigation of the children in the public schools and the analysis of some of those data. Mrs. Carlyle R. Hayes was of great help in the studies of young children at Woods Hole, Massachusetts.

already seen that fourteen of the seventy young delinquents showed the atypical stimulus-governed behavior.

If one compares in our delinquent and non-delinquent population of comparable age those who are not stimulus-governed ($N = 56$ and 59), one finds the following evidence indicating that the delinquents predominate at the reduction end of the perceptual reactance spectrum, although they do not fill it (see Fig. 25):

	Delinquents		Non-Delinquents	
	N	Percent	N	Percent
More pronounced reduction (Average of 6 mm or more)	17	33.6	7	11.8
Extremely pronounced reduction (Average of 12 mm or more)	4	7.14	0	0
Reducing by more than 12 mm with further stimulation (of 130 secs)	3	5.36	0	0
More pronounced augmentation (Average of 6 mm or more)	6	10.7	18	30.5

It should be noted that the cutting lines we used for comparing the delinquent and non-delinquent groups contrasts the number who were reducing or augmenting by 6 mm or more on an average of 12 measurements. These cutting lines indicate more pronounced reduction or augmentation, as they are higher than the ones we have used for dividing the population of augmenters and reducers from the moderates (see chapter 1, footnote 6).

It thus was found that (1) juvenile delinquents were twice as likely to be pronounced reducers as were those in the control group; (2) conversely, controls were three times as likely as juvenile delinquents to be pronounced augmenters; and that (3) there was a subcategory of delinquents whose reduction was so extreme that no control subjects were comparable.[9]

The statistical analysis of these data indicates that the delinquent group contains significantly more pronounced reducers and also

[9] Since an extreme reducer decreases the size of the measured object by 50 per cent and an extreme augmenter increases it by 50 per cent, there is a threefold difference between these two. The contrast between the numbers of reducers and augmenters in the delinquent and normal groups and the degree of their reduction should be considered with the size of this difference in mind.

more extremely pronounced reducers, and significantly fewer pronounced augmenters than the non-delinquent one.

Supporting evidence of this relationship of perceptual reactance to delinquency has now been found by an independent investigator in another state. Lawrence Z. Freedman, Foundations' Fund Research Professor in Psychiatry at the University of Chicago Medical School, will shortly be publishing these findings.

So much for the position of the delinquents in the spectrum of perceptual reactance stretching from extreme reduction to extreme augmentation. There appears also to be a spectrum of vulnerability to confinement and isolation. Those most vulnerable to isolation are at the reducing end of the perceptual modulation continuum, whereas those least vulnerable are at the augmenting end. The delinquents tend toward the reducing end and away from the augmenting end of the perceptual modulation spectrum more than do the non-delinquents.

The delinquents are thus by no means immune to the vulnerabilities associated with the reducing characteristics, that is to say, to suffering from monotony, isolation, and enforced inactivity. For example, a delinquent girl, explaining her association with young people who had run afoul of the law, said she "hung around with those kids because they were always doing something. Regular people don't do nothing."

The position of the juvenile delinquent on the perceptual modulation spectrum only begins to tell the story, for it appears that environmental conditions can change their needs, and even a moderate or less pronounced reducer can be brought to the point of stress if his environment should fall below what may be called his sensory subsistence level. Indeed, given the nature of our urban culture and the conditions under which the vast majority of these delinquent children live, this lack might easily develop for all except the 10 per cent of augmenters in this group.[10]

[10] The difficulty of obtaining labor permits for young people discourages the kind of activity needed by the reducer. Indeed, the adolescent reducer will frequently leave school with lower grades than the average (see chapter 7) and find no legitimate substitute activity available to him. The average intelligence, however, did not differ appreciably in those delinquent reducers and augmenters on whom we were able to obtain Wechsler I.Q. scores:

	N	Full Scale I.Q.	Verbal Scale I.Q.	Performance Scale I.Q.
Reducers	22	97.7	98.0	97.0
Augmenters	13	101.3	99.7	101.5

Many other factors besides sensory lack are involved in delinquency. Nevertheless, it is of interest that in this research it became apparent that being "bored" frequently meant the condition of sensory insufficiency. It may, indeed, be as close an indication as we can get in colloquial speech. Alberto Moravia, for example, writes: "Boredom, for me, is really a sort of insufficiency or scantiness of reality."

One of the difficulties about this concept is the lack of words with which to describe the restlessness and loss of feeling of identity and loss of contact with reality of the person deprived of enough sensation. Perhaps Byron said it as well as it has been said: "The great object of life is sensation—to feel that we exist, even though in pain. It is this 'craving void' which drives us to gaming—to battle—to travel—to intemperate, but keenly felt pursuits of any description, whose principal attraction is the agitation inseparable from their accomplishment" (1899).

The resulting avidity of the juvenile delinquent for sensation more readily expresses itself in action than in thought—in action leading to input from the ears, from the eyes, from touch, and from the feeling of rapid motion.[11]

The Reducer's Difficulty in Learning Good Social Behavior

The learning of good social behavior—or for that matter, the booklearning taught in schools—is more efficaciously encouraged by reward than by fear of punishment. But the reducing delinquent requires greater rewards than the augmenter to gain equal driving power. Indeed, we may need to look with fresh eyes at the story of the prodigal son. Whenever these wrongdoers are behaving well, we may need to treat them like a prodigal son and be generous in our encouragement.

[11] Attention has been drawn to the frequency with which bedwetting occurs among delinquents (Michaels 1955). The explanations put forward lean heavily on conative deficiencies—a lack of will power in the delinquent. An alternative explanation in keeping with the findings on reduction of stimuli is that the cues providing information about bodily needs are muted and often missed. (Of course, it is also necessary to remember that an empty bladder provides less sensation than the partially full one; when the sensory input approaches insufficiency the habit might be built up for retaining the bladder content.)

We need to remember that for the reducing delinquent, great resistance to pain goes along with vulnerability to monotony and relative afferent isolation. A delinquent, for example, will come to the infirmary with severe wounds and burns and seem hardly to be affected. Delinquent girls who are most difficult to handle prior to labor are often models of fortitude on the delivery table. Tattooing is widely practiced even among the girls, and when, for one reason or another, they would like to be free of it, the painful process of having it removed is tolerated with equanimity.

A serious aspect of the reducer's tolerance for pain is that such tolerance may contribute to his lack of motivation in learning. Despite rewards being more effective than punishment in encouraging learning, much of what we learn is reinforced by the cessation of pain. The extreme reducer is at a disadvantage here, for the ending of a stress that is scarcely noticed encourages him but little. In other words, the usual reinforcements for social learning of all kinds are minimally effective in the reducer because he diminishes the impact of most punishments and, indeed, of rewards that are intended to reinforce such behavior.[12]

A Low Sensory-Subsistence Level—Some Implications

Another serious aspect of the reducer's tolerance for pain, in terms of society, is that he cannot empathize adequately with experiences that he does not share. The extreme reducer fails to understand suffering with pain and may inflict it with little compunction. On the other side of the coin, because pain is, after all, sensation and better than no sensation under circumstances of sensory starvation, the reducer may welcome it as the lesser evil. As mentioned in chapter 2, he will deliberately inflict pain on himself, particularly when in solitary confinement, carving his flesh and burning himself with cigarette ends. The severe whippings that have been abolished by humanitarian concern may, indeed, have caused less suffering and therefore less disruption to some of the reducing delinquent youngsters than does the solitary confinement that is now used as a punishment in the institutions where they are detained. A delin-

[12] Delinquents are reported to be less conditionable than the rest of the population (Frank 1961). It is perhaps to be expected that the reducer would be a poor subject for experimental conditioning because of his reduction of afferent input.

quent male reducer volunteered, "I'd rather be hit on the head with a hammer than locked up in isolation." A stimulus-governed delinquent, placed in solitary confinement for seven days, described how he banged with a spoon to make noise "so that he could keep his mind." The only delinquent who said he preferred being locked up in isolation to suffering physical pain was an augmenter. He said, "I like being locked up. It gives me time to think."

It would seem that the education of reducing delinquents and potential delinquents might make allowance for their vulnerabilities and strengths. They appear to need change, movement, and speed, actual rather than symbolic instruction, bright colors, music, and company. The fact that many of these delinquent youngsters come from deprived homes means that their needs are even greater than the needs of youngsters with similar perceptual reactance who are fortunate enough to have many activities like swimming, boating, club games, and traveling available to them as part of their birthright. Perhaps we need to become more understanding of the extreme reducer's need in an urban setting for powerful noise and movement—for rock and roll, for pals and speed. In Wordsworth's words, he appears to have a "raging thirst for outrageous stimulation."

An environment that is close to nature, with snowstorms and turbulent oceans, boats that have to be handled in a gale, and animals that have to be tamed, provides excellently for the needs of the reducer. Some of the most successful methods of rehabilitating juvenile delinquents have reintroduced the youngsters to the natural challenge of the physical environment from which they are so largely insulated in their urban setting.[13]

In the history of medicine it was easier to grasp the idea of a man being poisoned by something he had taken in than to understand the concept of vitamin deficiency—that a man could be sick because of what he had not taken in. Similarly, it is easier to comprehend suffering caused by pain, by something that impinges on the individual, than to understand that which is caused by the absence of sensation, the kind of suffering to which the reducer is prone.

---

[13] Although the research reported was carried out with delinquents of eighteen years or younger, its implications are not irrelevant to the consideration of adult delinquents.

THE PERCEPTUAL REACTANCE OF THE ALCOHOLIC

As shown in chapter 3, alcohol causes a dramatic alteration in the perceptual reactance at the augmenting end of the spectrum, while at the reducing end there is little alteration. Hence, it might be expected that the attraction of alcohol would be strongest for those who had experienced its greatest effects and that drinking to the point of addiction would be more likely to occur among the augmenters and moderates than among the reducers. The findings in our studies of alcoholics supports this hypothesis.

Our studies were made at the Boston Sanatorium with the co-operation of Dr. David Sherman, the superintendent, and Miss Gertrude Daly, his administrative assistant. The Sanatorium, originally intended for the treatment of tuberculosis, found so high a proportion of alcoholics among its recurring clientele that it turned to the treatment of their alcoholism as well as their tuberculosis. Indeed, the first halfway house in the country for the rehabilitation of those alcoholics who had been relieved of their tuberculosis was set up there.

The Study of Alcoholic Patients

One study was made of fifteen alcoholic patients each of whom was well enough to be seen for two long sessions. Both large-block and small-block stimulation were used. (Six other patients had to be excluded from this study because they were drinking in the hospital and their condition on the days of testing could not be ascertained with assurance, but we will return later to their contribution.) A second much briefer study of twenty-five alcoholics was completed but as these patients were not well enough to take part in the investigations in the laboratory, the work had to be limited to scores on the Maudsley Personality Inventory and interviews conducted while the patients were in bed. All patients with a neurological or psychiatric condition other than that of alcoholism were excluded from both studies.

Of the fifteen patients in the first study, one was strongly stimulus-governed and two others showed milder stimulus-governed scores. The patients showing this atypical perceptual style turned out to have serious behavior problems in addition to their alcoholism; one of them, for example, had been before a court of law on more than one occasion, charged with assault.

Of the remaining alcoholic patients, half were augmenters and half were moderates; none were reducers. Moreover, all of the moderates were augmenting slightly.

These fifteen alcoholics were compared with the normal group of twenty-three subjects used in the study of the effect of alcohol on whom only scores for large-block stimulation had been collected. The reducing tendency of the alcoholics, as shown on large-block scores, was significantly less than that of the normal group: -0.33 as compared with -3.30. (The Mann-Whitney U-test was utilized.)

In addition, the total augmentation-reduction score, as displayed on both the large- and small-block stimulation sessions, was calculated. These scores were compared with those of a group of thirty-three students whose large- and small-block stimulation scores were also obtained. Again the alcoholics showed the significantly greater augmenting tendencies.

One of the difficulties about studying these addicts is that if one has collected a really good sample of alcoholics, the likelihood exists that these patients will make every effort to obtain a drink, whatever may be the rules of the investigation or of the institution where they are temporarily confined. Being aware of this danger, the nurses and physicians were asked to report to the investigator any patient who was found to have been "drinking on the wards," as the saying goes in this hospital. Such patients were excluded from the study as the risk was great that they had been under the influence of alcohol when tested, in which case the perceptual reactance scores obtained on them would have been likely to be false, in that they would show the reduction induced by the alcohol.

Two of the six alcoholics who had been excluded from the study because they had been drinking while the study was in progress had reducing scores. (One of these patients was reported by the nurse in January to have been "drunk every day since Thanksgiving.") The remaining four patients had augmenting or moderate scores. So that even if the six patients who were suspected of drinking during the testing period had been included in the sample of alcoholics, the total alcoholic group would nevertheless show significantly more augmentation than a comparable non-alcoholic one.

Alcoholic Scores on the Maudsley Personality Inventory

The twenty-five alcoholic patients who were given the Maudsley Personality Inventory showed significantly lower extraversion scores than the fifty non-alcoholic patients in the same hospital with whom they were compared. It will be remembered that in the discussion of the Maudsley Personality Inventory in chapter 2 we found that low extraversion scores are associated with the augmenting perceptual reactance and were found in persons who were intolerant of pain.

The danger of addiction to alcohol appears thus to be greatest at the augmenting end of the spectrum, according to these investigations. The risk seems to be great in those who suffer much from the bombardment of the perceptual environment.[14] Alcohol subdues their experiences—those that are pleasant as well as those that are unpleasant. The fact that "ecstasy is deeper than heartache" may, in part, protect the fortunately vast numbers of non-alcoholic augmenters from using this form of escape from their sensibility.

The Contrasted Perceptual Modulation of Alcoholics and Juvenile Delinquents

The alcoholics, as we have seen, appear to occupy the augmenting end of the spectrum and the juvenile delinquents seem to occupy the reducing end, although the overlap is considerable, particularly among the moderates. There also appear to be many fewer stimulus-governed persons among alcoholics than among juvenile delinquents. There are thus some contrasts in the perceptual modulation of these two groups. It is to be expected, therefore, that there will also be contrasts in their vulnerabilities during the pre-delinquent and the pre-alcoholic phases of their lives. These differences underline the varied prophylactic measures likely to be needed to combat these two very different problems.

[14] Alcoholics, like delinquents, are, of course, a heterogeneous group. Heavy drinkers may be even more varied. For example, the man who gets drunk to create a disturbance is not likely to be an augmenter. He is prone to be a spree-drinker and hence does not become an alcoholic as frequently as the persistent heavy drinker.

Perceptual Modulation and
6 Cigarette Smoking

Make it thy business to know thyself.

MIGUEL DE CERVANTES (1547)

CIGARETTE SMOKING

A small pilot study on cigarette smoking provides one example of how information about perceptual modulation can throw added light on a practical problem.

Those perceptual modulation types who are minimally sensitive to pain and discomfort tend to be less concerned about health and more readily take health hazards.[1] The association between ill-health and smoking has been increasingly pointed out in recent years. People are warned that the heavy smoker is more likely to develop heart conditions, cancer, and other pathology. Does the smoking behavior in general suggest that reducers are actually less affected by such warnings than augmenters? There is some slight evidence now that this is so.

The Relevance of the Reducers Tolerance of Discomfort

One might predict that the reducer's insensitivity to discomfort would increase his tolerance for the throat irritations and other discomforts that interfere sufficiently with the pleasure of some smokers to make them limit the amount they smoke. Some investigators attribute the relationship between smoking and lung cancer to the factor of chronic irritation. It is not improbable that the

---

[1] The relevant findings about the health behavior of reducers were reported and discussed in chapter 2.

reducer's insensitivity to discomfort may often lead him to ignore such potentially dangerous irritation until it does become chronic.

Smoking and Additional Sensory Input

From the findings, it would appear that cigarette smoking may be contributing to the compensation for the lower sensory subsistence threshold of persons in a state of reduction. In our results, as we would expect, the reducers were more avid than the augmenters for a socially-acceptable source of self-determined sensory input that provides contact for the lips, mouth, and fingers where sensitivity is great, and that adds sensations of smell, taste, and warmth for good measure. This association may be particularly interesting to those engaged in cancer prevention and the question of why people find smoking cigarettes so satisfying an activity.

Individual Differences in Smoking

In our study of delinquents it was found that the age at which these adolescents reported that they started to smoke is significantly younger for the reducers than it is for the augmenters. More reducers were smoking by the age of twelve. Moreover, when asked about enjoyment of smoking, no reducer said that he did not enjoy smoking very much, whereas 50 per cent of the augmenters reported their lack of enthusiasm for this activity.

Another item of interest is that 40 per cent of the reducers and no augmenters said that they expected to smoke more in five years time than they do now. None of the reducers stopped smoking after having started, but 12 per cent of the augmenters ceased to smoke; and 40 per cent of the reducers and only 12 per cent of the augmenters made no attempt to stop smoking. In addition, in a group of twenty-nine adult women there were significantly more smokers among the reducers than among the augmenters (71 per cent as against 40 per cent). The smoking trends of the reducer were also supported by the findings in a small group of Cambridge school children (see Table 14).[2]

[2] Of course there will be many exceptions to the smoking trends among reducers. For example, there is evidence that certain kinds of athletes, those doing "contact" activities, come from the reducing end of the perceptual modulation spectrum (see chapter 7). In their training, avoidance of smoking is often greatly stressed. Concern with athletic achievements may lead these reducers to limit the amount smoked.

TABLE 14

SOME DIFFERENCES IN CIGARETTE SMOKING

Name of Group		Augmenters Per Cent	Reducers Per Cent
Male delinquents	Report that they started smoking at age twelve or younger	0 (N = 8)	50 (N = 10) *ᵃ
Male delinquents	Report that they do not enjoy smoking very much	50 (N = 8)	0 (N = 10) *ᵃ
Adult women	Report that they smoke	36 (N = 11)	82 (N = 11) *ᵃ
Cambridge public school children	Report that they smoke	9 (N = 11)	40 (N = 5) ᵃ

* Significant at .05 level for a one-tail test.
ᵃ Exact probability test.

Further support for these findings comes from the characteristics reported in the literature of differences between the heavy smoker and the non-smoker, for some of these differences are similar to those between the reducer and the augmenter. (Heath 1958; McArthur, Waldron, and Dickinson 1958; Eysenck et al. 1960; Eysenck 1962.)

These results about reduction, augmentation, and sensory input apply to behavior under normal conditions. When, however, a pronounced loss of environmental stimulation occurs, the moderate, and even the augmenter, may also search for controlled amounts of sensory input. Thus, it is of particular interest that those who are unemployed and those who have lost their mates show a higher consumption of cigarettes (Haenzel, Shimkin, and Miller 1956; Matarazzo and Saslow 1960).

Observers have noted time and again that there is an association between the smoking of cigarettes and the drinking of alcohol (Heath 1958; McArthur, Waldron, and Dickinson 1958; Matarazzo and Saslow 1960). Alcohol alters perceptual style; as we have seen, its consumption is followed by increased reduction, the state that increases a person's need for sensory input. Thus, one would expect that the self-determined increments of sensory input from cigarette smoking would be particularly acceptable after the drinking of alcohol.

We do *not* know as yet the effect of nicotine on perceptual modulation. When we do, we may understand better the examples of excessive smoking to be found at the augmenting end of the spectrum.[3]

These preliminary findings on the relationship between cigarette smoking, sensitivity to pain or discomfort, and perceptual style are reinforced by the fact that they all point in the same direction. What is evident, but should be emphasized in terms of preventive medicine, is that prophylactic health measures seem least likely to be taken by those whose behavior indicates that they are the ones in whom to expect a high incidence of health hazards, as is shown schematically in Table 15.

TABLE 15

DIFFERENCES BETWEEN PERSONS IN A STATE OF REDUCTION AND THOSE IN A STATE OF AUGMENTATION THAT MAY BE RELATED TO THEIR HEALTH

PERSONS IN A STATE OF REDUCTION	PERSONS IN A STATE OF AUGMENTATION
Least sensitive to danger signs of pain and discomfort	Most sensitive to danger signs of pain and discomfort
Need more sensory input	Need less sensory input
Most neglect of prophylactic health measures	Least neglect of prophylactic health measures
Least concerned with problems of health	Most concerned with problems of health
Start to smoke cigarettes earlier in life	Start to smoke cigarettes later in life
Greatest difficulty in stopping smoking	Least difficulty in stopping smoking
Smoke more cigarettes	Smoke fewer cigarettes

[3] We know that sensory stimulation decreases augmentation at the augmenting end of the spectrum. Does cigarette smoking provide sufficient stimulation for the augmenter to be temporarily freed from sensory bombardment which he may be experiencing as excessive? The possibility that the augmenter uses cigarette smoking as "fine tuning" to cut out some sensory distractions would seem worth exploring further.

Some Speculations on the
7 Import of these Findings

I have put on these masks to show you my face.
                                    MAURICE ENGLISH (1963)

Individual differences in suffering was the original interest and the recurrent theme of the research forming the basis of this volume. Varied reactions to physical pain have, of course, long been noted and the assumption had been made previously that these variations were largely due to differences in the self-control of the patient, in the reassurance available to him, and in variation in the cultural mores. Our research suggests, however, that these differences may, in part, be due to ways of *experiencing* the environment that vary according to the perceptual modulation of the individual. Moreover, subdued experience in a state of reduction and intense experience in a state of augmentation may affect a person's suffering from different kinds of distress.

Other Differences between Reducers and Augmenters

The extreme differences in sensibility between the augmenter and reducer lead one to expect many other differences between them. For example, since activity arouses sensation, one could predict greater activity in the reducer. He might be likely to prefer having many friends, whereas fewer, perhaps deeper, friendships would be more characteristic of the augmenter. The reducer might wish for an occupation bringing him into contact with many other people, while the augmenter would wish to work alone.

Here follow a few scattered findings that lend some support to these suppositions. They reach the requisite levels of significance although involving very small samples and are included only in the hope of stimulating further research into differences in personality that accompany variation in perceptual reactance.

The assessment of the male delinquents by counselors who were in constant contact with them was part of a routine procedure at the institutions where we received cooperation in carrying out the studies described in chapter 5. Counselors were unaware of our findings about the perceptual characteristics of these boys. In the reports of the counselors, the reducers were described as active, as participating in all activities and in sports more frequently than the augmenters. The augmenters were described as quiet and inactive, avoiding activities more frequently than the reducers (see Table 16).

Some additional findings about the greater activity and the tolerance for pain at the reducing end of the perceptual modulation spectrum in contrast to the augmenting end were collected at the University of California. This research, carried out by Dean Ryan and his associates, compared the reduction and tolerance for pain of three groups: those who chose athletic activities, such as wrestling and football, which involved physical contact; those who chose athletic activities, such as tennis or golf, which did not involve physical contact; and those who did not take part in any athletics and did not wish to do so. In their group of 60 subjects, the degree of perceptual reduction was greatest among the 20 "contact"-athletic students and least among the 20 non-athletic students. The degree of reduction of the 20 "non-contact" athletic students lay between these two extremes.

Tolerance for pain was found to be greatest in the contact-athletic students who showed the greatest reduction and least in the non-athletic students, who showed the least reduction. Medium pain tolerance was found in the non-contact athletic students, who also showed medium reduction. The difference was significant at the .005 level for both perceptual reduction and pain tolerance in comparing the contact-athletic students with the non-athletic students (Ryan and Kovacic 1966; Ryan and Foster 1966).

In reporting to us about their personal relationships in answer to standardized questions about how many close boy friends and how many close girl friends each had, the reducers stated, in contrast to the augmenters, that they had ten or more close boy friends and also ten or more close girl friends (see Table 16).

TABLE 16

Some Additional Characteristics That Differ in the
Reducer and the Augmenter

Name of Group		Augmenters Per Cent	Reducers Per Cent
Male delinquents	Described by supervisors as: participating in sports, active and participating in all activities	16 ($N = 13$)	55 ($N = 22$) *b
Male delinquents	Described by supervisors as: quiet, inactive, lazy, and avoiding activities	62 ($N = 13$)	9 ($N = 22$) ***b
Male delinquents	Report that they have ten or more close boy friends	33 ($N = 9$)	81 ($N = 11$) *a
Male delinquents	Report that they have ten or more close girl friends	0 ($N = 9$)	45 ($N = 11$) *a
Cambridge public school children	Average school grades	77.9 ($N = 9$)	66.9 ($N = 5$) ***c
Adult women	Report that they would like to have nine or more hours of sleep at night	50 ($N = 8$)	8 ($N = 12$) a
Adult women	Report that they would like to have six or less hours of sleep at night	0 ($N = 8$)	33 ($N = 12$) a
Male delinquents	Report that they bite their nails	20 ($N = 5$)	63 ($N = 8$) a

* Significant at the .05 level for a one-tail test.
** Significant at the .01 level for a one-tail test.
*** Significant at the .005 level for a one-tail test.
a Exact probability test.
b Chi-square test.
c Mann-Whitney U-test.

The contrast between reducers and augmenters in their sensory needs and vulnerabilities makes it of interest that there appeared to be a shortage of augmenters among the expectant mothers coming to the obstetric department at Beth Israel Hospital to have their babies, as well as among the mothers of illegitimate babies at Tewksbury Hospital.[1] Moreover, the two most unusually extreme

[1] The bulk of the findings about perceptual reduction and augmentation are based on the normal population. Atypical and pathological groups were also studied as they may provide valuable additional information.

augmenters in the adult group were both found to have almost no sex life.

School grades are, to a certain extent, dependent on one's willingness to cultivate the talents associated with language. In such cultivation, a person who is willing to spend a great deal of time sitting still while reading or listening and who, moreover, is content to deal with symbols rather than realities, has advantages. These characteristics appear to be those which we find in the augmenter rather than in the reducer. Thus, other things being equal, one might expect that an augmenter would have better school grades than does a reducer, and that is what was found in one small group—the Cambridge public school children—from whom we were able to collect school grades. The augmenters have the highest grades, the reducers the lowest and the moderates fall between; the difference between reducers and augmenters reaches the .009 level of probability.[2] We found the same trend of lower scholastic grades for reducers among student nurses at Beth Israel Hospital's School of Nursing.

According to augmentation-reduction theory, the augmenter, during his waking hours, is having a richer perceptual life than the reducer.[3] One might, therefore, expect that the augmenter would require longer periods of recuperation than the reducer and that this contrast would be noticeable in differences in their wishes for sleep. One might also venture the additional query whether the "emptiness" of sleep might not be welcomed by the augmenter but constitute something of a threat to the reducer.

Providing some support for these hypotheses, we found differences in attitude toward sleeping in one normal adult female group of twenty subjects, members of the nursing staff at Beth Israel Hospital. More augmenters than reducers stated that they would

---

[2] In the study of the public school children, the figures were collected by Jacob Schonfield of the University of Maryland while he was at the City of Cambridge Department of Health. Betsy Abrams, Connie Gaetz, and Kathleen O'Brien helped with the testing in some of the other studies, to each of whom I am indebted.

[3] In his sixth year, a young augmenter had the following conversation with his mother:

Boy: "Mummy, do you know you're almost beautiful."
Mother: "I am sorry I am not completely beautiful—if that would please you."
Boy: "Oh, no, I wouldn't like that at all. There would be too much gold and color about."

like nine or more hours of sleep each night, while more reducers than augmenters would prefer to have six hours sleep or less (see Table 16).

Again, reasoning from the greater need of the reducer to garner sensation, we predicted that nail biting would occur with greater frequency in the reducer than in the augmenter. We obtained some data on nail biting in a delinquent group and this difference was borne out (see Table 16).

Psychosomatic Medicine and Reduction and Augmentation

Speculation about some matters that have not yet been experimentally verified may spur others to go further with this research. That

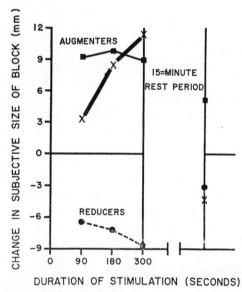

Fig. 26. Photophobic boy, effect of stimulation with large and small blocks (x━x), combined means.

the different kinds of resistance possessed by the reducer and augmenter may lead to different types of problems in clinical medicine in these two perceptual styles was suggested by the findings reported in chapter 2. The extreme augmenter in Figure 26, for instance, is a boy with photophobia without any known pathology—that is to say, he experiences discomfort from the presence of light of an intensity that leaves most persons reasonably undisturbed. In contrast, the extreme reducer in Figure 10 is an adult male with a peptic ulcer, who experienced no pain from his ulceration.[4]

It seems likely that different problems will also be presented in psychosomatic medicine and psychiatry by those at opposite ends of the spectrum of subdued and intense experience. Physiological changes accompany emotions. These physiological changes cause the person who, for example, is afraid, to report sensations ranging from dryness of his mouth to his "hair standing on end." If these sensations are reduced in some persons and augmented in others, "psychic" fear might also be found to differ in quality depending on the perceptual modulation occurring. (Indeed, one school of thought holds that the feeling of fear results from the sensations following upon such physiological changes.) That is to say, reduction and augmentation of the internal cues accompanying emotions may be contributing in part to the differences between persons in their reactions to these emotions. Extreme augmentation of the internal cues accompanying emotions could contribute in part to the development of some psychiatric symptoms.

Perceptual modulation is clearly not a conscious process. The person showing reduction or augmentation is not aware of any processing of the sensations he receives.

Augmentation and Reduction in Relation to the Central Nervous System

Since auditory bombardment causes a change in kinesthetic augmentation, it appears that the central nervous system, at some

---

[4] The degree of augmentation and reduction of the male patient presented in Figure 26 is shown against the background of the normal population of reducers and augmenters in Figure 3. On the whole, the most extreme examples of augmentation and reduction seem to occur in males. It may be that there are biological advantages in limiting the number of females who are oversensitive to pain and to the other pronounced stimulation that the bearing and rearing of children involves. At the other extreme of perceptual modulation, the successful care of children might be hindered if a mother were too insensitive to their needs.

One other suggestive sex characteristic found was a tendency for females to show an increase in stimulus-governed trends in the last few days before a menstrual period, and possibly also during the last weeks of pregnancy.

point in or above the brain stem, must be involved in the process. It does not necessarily follow that the central mechanism is always involved when a change in augmentation or reduction occurs; nevertheless, one should, in this connection, take note of another clinical example of an association between augmentation and tolerance for pain that appears to involve the central nervous system. The pain of a phantom limb that occurs when a real limb is absent is usually considered to be central in origin. A severe case of such pain in an extreme augmenter was described in chapter 1.

It is, moreover, clear that when increased tolerance for pain of central origin, such as that from a phantom limb, is achieved by the use of aspirin, for example, the diminished augmentation accompanying the administration of this drug must be thought of as acting centrally; otherwise, the change in tolerance would not occur. At our present stage of knowledge about perceptual reduction and augmentation, perhaps the most helpful neurological model of these processes is to think of them as contrasted examples of the central modulation of sensory perception. Such central modulation may be dependent on the presence and nature of reverberating circuits in the nervous system (Livingston 1943).

Biochemical factors undoubtedly will be found to play an important part in perceptual modulation. For example, Robert Henkin and his colleagues of the National Institutes of Health at Bethesda, Maryland, have recently demonstrated that non-psychiatric medical patients with untreated adrenal cortical insufficiencies, such as Addison's disease, show characteristic sensory phenomena including extreme perceptual reduction. (Henkin et al. 1963 and 1966). Silverman reports that these patients show no overlap with a "normal" control group and that correction of the adrenal cortical deficiency brings perceptual reduction within the normal range (Silverman 1966). Our study of female students at Wellesley College suggests that an increase in atypical perceptual modulation occurs during premenstrual days. Moreover, there was suggestive evidence in another study of expectant mothers, before and after the birth of their babies, that aberrations of perceptual modulation accompany some pregnancies. Here changes in steroid hormones are the common factor in that they occur premenstrually, during pregnancy and in association with adrenal cortical insufficiency. In addition there have been shown to be disturbances in steroid metabolism associated with some forms of schizophrenia. The evidence for atypical perceptual responses in schizophrenic patients was discussed in chapter 4.[5]

It seems highly likely from fragments of information now available that a person's basic perceptual reactance pattern will be shown to be partially genetically determined. Predisposition in one or the other direction, however, probably can be greatly altered by environmental conditions. Temporary alterations in perceptual reactance were shown, for example, to follow upon sensory bombardment; moreover, there were perceptual characteristics in the group who were born deaf, suggesting that a less temporary adaptation away from the reduction end of the continuum had taken place in them.

The Spectrum from Subdued to Intense Experience

More than one hundred years ago, E. H. Weber wrote about the consciousness of self: "The sum, the unsorted chaos of sensations from all the sensitive parts of the body, which leads to the consciousness of self" (Weber 1851). Everything that has come out of this research suggests that the sum of such sensations is diminished for the reducer and increased for the augmenter. That under these circumstances the reducer might appear greedy for sensations does not strain our understanding, nor is it difficult to comprehend the possibility of his diminished consciousness of self and consciousness of the persons with whom he relates.

The augmenter, in contrast to the reducer, appears to have intense consciousness of himself and of others. Into his mouth perhaps we may properly put Shakespeare's phrase, "I could be bounded in a nutshell and count myself a king of infinite space." A part of this capacity may lie in the augmenter's rich inner life, a mirror of the richness coming into him from the environment. In addition, his independence from sensory want frees him to cultivate his own mind.

The most effective way of demonstrating variation in perceptual modulation is to examine the extremes of the distribution where the contrasts are clearest. Our resultant preoccupation with the reducer and augmenter should not be interpreted as implying that the moderate is of minor importance. We saw, for example, in

[5] The earlier studies of Wertheimer and Wertheimer (1954) and Wertheimer (1955) are of interest in this connection.

chapter 2, that he was moderately tolerant of the stresses of pain and of isolation and restriction of activity. With an environment that varies from providing over-much sensory stimulation to threatening to fall below the sensory subsistence level, the moderate may be the best equipped to cope. In contemporary cultures such an environment appears to occur frequently.

What all this means, nevertheless, is that the concept of the strong man who can stand up to any type of great stress seems to be erroneous. The findings suggest that there are different kinds of strength and different kinds of stress to which some perceptual modulation types, but not others, are vulnerable.

One wonders about the biological functions of the varieties of perceptual modulation and the associated differences of strength and vulnerability. It may be that the reducer and the augmenter represent varied kinds of adaptation to a world in which optimal conditions occur for the survival of each of these perceptual styles.

The association of human beings in civilization's communal enterprise may need both those whose perceptual modulation encourages them to delve deeply and those others who spread themselves thin and wide. The availability of persons of such different capacities furnishes strength to the social organization. For these capacities to function at their optimum it would seem, from the knowledge now available, highly desirable that each person comes to regard himself as the guardian of the different vulnerabilities of the other. But the success of these differences in personal constitution depends most certainly upon a clear recognition of the role that they play. At present we are still at the beginning of understanding the nature and usefulness of these fundamental differences.

Appendix A

Instructions for the Kinesthetic Determination of the Extent of Reduction and Augmentation [1]

OUTLINE OF CONTENTS

Introduction

The tester should be able to move smoothly during the whole procedure. Practice and familiarity with the equipment are essen-

[1] The instructions in this Appendix were originally issued over the names of the present author and Mrs. T. Holland. Mrs. Holland drew all the illustrations and used this guide with many persons being trained to carry out investigations with these techniques. She has also made a number of valuable contributions to other aspects of this work.

tial. Some confusion may result from the complexity of the procedure.

Ordinarily the tester should commence by reading the entire text
with care, frequently referring to the description and the illustra-
tion of the equipment (Fig. 27) and to the summary in Section F.

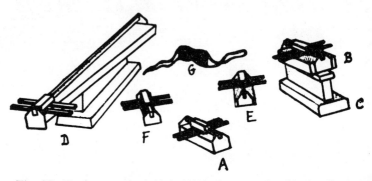

Fig. 27. Equipment used: (*a*) 1½-inch measuring block; (*b*) 2½-
inch stimulating block; (*c*) stand for stimulating and measuring blocks;
(*d*) tapered block; (*e*) 2-inch measuring block; (*f*) 1-inch stimulating
block; (*g*) blindfold.

Subsequently the tester will proceed to a more detailed study of
special sections of the text.

A. ASPECTS THAT WILL INVALIDATE THE INVESTIGATION

1. Do not test a subject after any drug or alcohol has been taken,
   after he has been exposed to considerable heat or cold or any
   excessive stimulation, for example, bathing, ironing, typing in
   an office where many other machines are being used, or the
   prolonged sound of a pneumatic drill, or when he is greatly
   fatigued. Do not test a subject when he is feeling sick—even if
   he says he only has a "cold."

   When you are attempting to obtain a "normal" population
   sample, be sure to exclude all subjects in whom—after suitable
   questioning—you obtain any evidence of psychiatric, neurological (e.g., history of concussion), or endocrinological conditions.

   As there are changes in perceptual modulation within the
   menstrual cycle, make sure that the testing sessions are close

together or, should this prove impossible, that they take place during comparable phases of the cycle, and never during the week preceding its onset.

2. During the three-quarters of an hour resting period, permit no smoking, and no excessive stimulation of any other kind (sound, light, heat, cold, and so forth).

3. At no time allow the subject to see the testing equipment. The tester must take care to refer to the blocks in these words: "another block," "a different block," and so forth; *never:* "The first block," "the same block," and so forth.

B. EQUIPMENT

The equipment consists of a box containing:

1. One long tapered block of wood. It is called the tapered block and is used only in conjunction with the measuring block. The tapered block is used in the subject's left hand so that he can indicate the width of the measuring block in his right hand. (This position is reversed for left-handed subjects.) Running the length of the block, which is 30 inches long, is a ruler marked in 1 inch and also ⅛ inch and mounted around the ruler is a pair of parallel sticks used for finger guides. (See Fig. 27 above.) The block tapers from ½ inch at its narrow end to 4 inches at its wide end.

2. Four rectangular blocks measuring 1, 1½, 2 and 2½ inches in width. Each of these blocks is 6 inches long and is equipped with finger guides. These four rectangular blocks are the stimulating and measuring blocks.[2]

3. One stand to act as a base for the four rectangular blocks whenever they are in use.

4. One blindfold, stopwatch, pad of paper, and pen.

C. LARGE-BLOCK AND SMALL-BLOCK STIMULATION TESTS

Two tests are administered with the equipment described. Both of these tests are given to the subject, but they must be separated by a 48-hour interval. The procedure for giving both the large-block

[2] We have been experimenting with smaller blocks for young children to meet the size of their handspan. (See chapter 5, footnote 5.)

and the small-block stimulation tests is identical, except for the sizes of the rectangular blocks used for stimulation and measurement.

In the large-block stimulation test, the largest block, measuring 2½ inches in width, is used for stimulation, and the 1½ inch block is used for measurement. In the small-block stimulation test, the smallest block, 1 inch in width, is used for stimulation, and the 2-inch block is used for measurement.[3]

The block is always held between the fingers of the subject's right hand, unless he is left-handed. (If the subject is left-handed, the tapered block is on the right, and stimulating and measuring blocks are held in the left hand.)

The function of the tapered block is to enable the subject to indicate to the tester, with his left hand, the width of the block in his right hand.

D. PROCEDURE

The test is divided into four parts.

1. *The 45-minute rest.*

Every subject must rest both of his hands for 45 minutes before the test is given. The tester should take particular care that nothing touches the balls of the index finger and thumb of either hand during this rest period (see Fig. 28). During this rest period the tester should find out whether the subject is left-handed.[4]

---

[3] See Summary at end of this Appendix.

[4] The left-handed subjects should be considered as a separate group, as the degree of dominance of the opposite side of their brain is *not* a mirror-image of that in a right-handed person.

To determine handedness, we have been asking the subject to try and touch a pencil that is held out of reach, centrally above and to the front of his head (approximately 18 inches above and 18 inches in front of the top of his head). This is repeated 3 times. Then he is asked to try and touch a watch that is placed out of reach on the table (on a line that passes through the subject's midline). This is also repeated 3 times. The subject is scored in terms of the proportion of times the right hand is used. After completion of these six trials the subject is asked whether he regards himself as right- or left-handed.

While the trials for handedness are taking place, the subject sits with his arms symmetrically placed on the table. During the remainder of the time, in order to avoid the fatigue caused by maintaining a constant position, the position of the hands, elbows, and arms may be changed at will.

2. *The test.*

The subject, after resting his hands, is seated at a table large enough for the equipment. The tester blindfolds the subject before placing the equipment on the table. The long tapered block is placed by the subject's left hand, with the narrow end toward the subject. The measuring block is set on the stand and placed by the subject's right hand. Figure 29 shows a top view of the proper angles and position of blocks in relation to the

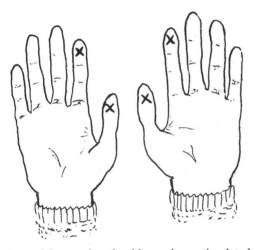

Fig. 28. Area of fingers that should remain unstimulated during rest periods.

subject; and this position should be maintained for the periods of measurement. It is suggested that the table be marked so as to ensure this constant position.

Taking care not to touch the subject's fingers, the tester lifts the subject's right hand (see Fig. 30), and places his fingers in position between the finger guides on the measuring block (see Fig. 31).

The tester must repeatedly check the subject's fingers to be sure they are touching the block.

The tester now indicates, by sliding the subject's hand, that the sides are parallel. The tester then places the subject's left hand on the narrow end of the tapered block (see Fig. 32).

The subject's arms must be above the table—*not* resting on it.

The subject's thumb and index finger are between the finger guides, and the tester slides the subject's hand toward the wider

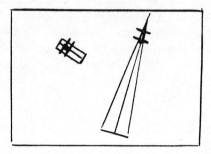

Fig. 29. Position of tapered block and measuring block on table.

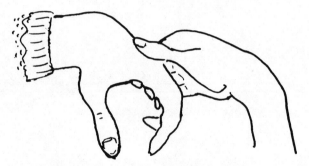

Fig. 30. Guiding the subject's hands.

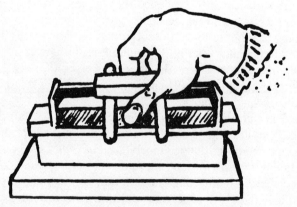

Fig. 31. Position of fingers on measuring block (side view).

end of the block so that the subject can feel that the block tapers. The tester must take care not to slide the guide beyond the 8-inch reading on the tapered block. The hand is then returned all the way to the narrow end of the block (the end nearest the subject) and must always be in this position at the beginning of measuring.

The tester asks the subject to find with his left hand on the tapered block the place that feels to him just as wide as the

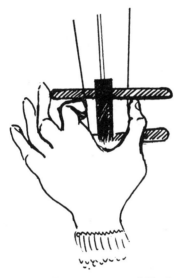

Fig. 32. Position of fingers on tapered block (top view).

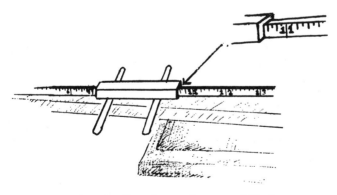

Fig. 33. The ruler on the tapered block.

measuring block between the fingers of his right hand. The tester then reads the position reached by the front end of the central finger guide on the ruler and records this number to the nearest ⅛ in. as the first baseline measurement (see Fig. 33).

The subject now slides his hand back to the narrow end of the tapered block and makes another measurement. Altogether the tester records six successive baseline measurements (see Table 17). The finger guide must always be returned to the narrow end of the tapered block between measurements.

The subject must be told to say "here" when he has found the size that feels equivalent, and he must hold his fingers in place for a moment until the measurement can be recorded.

TABLE 17

COMMENCEMENT OF A RECORD
(LARGE-BLOCK STIMULATION)

Series of Measurements	Practice Trials		(1)	(2)	(3)	(4)
I (Baseline)	(11⅞)	(12⅜)	14⅞	14⅝	14⅞	14⅝
II (After 90 seconds stimulation) III (After 180 seconds stimulation) IV (After 300 seconds stimulation)						
Rest Period						
V (After 15-minute rest period)						

The tester then removes the subject's left hand from the tapered block and guides it to a position, palm upwards, on the table, instructing the subject to let the hand rest in this position. The tester next tells the subject to keep his fingers on the block in his right hand. Then the tester and the subject lift the measuring block off the stand and the tester rapidly places the stimulating block on the stand. The block and its stand are moved to a position roughly parallel to the edge of the table, a position which is less fatiguing for the subject. This position is, however, used *only* during the stimulating period.

The tester next removes the subject's right hand from the measuring block and places it on the stimulating block, instructing him to rub the block by sliding his fingers along its whole length, backwards and forwards, at any rate he likes, until he is told to stop. The total time of this first stimulation period is 90 seconds.

Immediately following the 90 seconds of rubbing, the tester lifts the stimulating block from the stand and, while the subject's fingers remain on the stimulating block, the tester replaces the measuring block on the stand and returns block and stand to original position for measuring. The tester again places subject's right hand on the measuring block and his left hand on the long tapered block and asks him to find the place on the tapered block that feels the same as the width of the measuring block. This value is recorded and three more measurements are then made and recorded.

The subject's left hand is again rested and his right hand stimulated as before by rubbing for 90 seconds. After this stimulation, four more measurements are made. The subject then rubs the stimulating block for 120 seconds. Four more measurements are made and recorded. This completes the second part of the procedure, and the tester should now have 18 recorded numbers (see Table 18).

TABLE 18

CONTINUATION OF A RECORD OF MEASUREMENTS
(LARGE-BLOCK STIMULATION)

Series of Measurements	Practice Trials		(1)	(2)	(3)	(4)
I (Baseline)	(11⅞)	(12⅜)	14²⁄₈	14⁴⁄₈	14²⁄₈	14⁶⁄₈
II (After 90-second stimulation)			12⁶⁄₈	13²⁄₈	13⁴⁄₈	14
III (After 180-second stimulation)			11	13²⁄₈	12²⁄₈	12⁷⁄₈
IV (After 300-second stimulation)			9²⁄₈	10⁴⁄₈	11⁴⁄₈	12⁴⁄₈
Rest Period						
V (After 15-minute rest period)						

The tester then removes all equipment from the table and takes off the subject's blindfold, instructing him to continue to keep both hands from touching anything.

3. *The 15-minute rest.*

The subject now rests his hands as before for 15 minutes. The tester then replaces the blindfold and puts the equipment back on the table in position for measuring.

4. *Measurement after the rest period.*

The tester now places the subject's hands in position for measuring and again reads and records four measurements. This is the end of the test period, and the equipment must all be removed from the table before the subject's blindfold is taken off. The tester should now have 22 numbers recorded on his sheet (see Table 19).

TABLE 19

COMPLETED RECORD OF A REDUCER
(LARGE-BLOCK STIMULATION)

Series of Measurements	Practice Trials		(1)	(2)	(3)	(4)
I (Baseline)	$(11\frac{7}{8})$	$(12\frac{3}{8})$	$14\frac{2}{8}$	$14\frac{4}{8}$	$14\frac{2}{8}$	$14\frac{6}{8}$
II (After 90-second stimulation)			$12\frac{6}{8}$	$13\frac{2}{8}$	$13\frac{4}{8}$	14
III (After 180-second stimulation)			11	$13\frac{2}{8}$	$12\frac{3}{8}$	$12\frac{7}{8}$
IV (After 300-second stimulation)			$9\frac{2}{8}$	$10\frac{4}{8}$	$11\frac{4}{8}$	$12\frac{4}{8}$
Rest Period						
V (After 15-minute rest period)			$10\frac{3}{8}$	11	$11\frac{3}{8}$	$12\frac{1}{8}$

The subject should be tested again after a 48-hour period or more has elapsed. In order to avoid possible diurnal variations the tester should schedule the subject's tests for the same hour of the day as the initial test, but not too late in the day when the subject may be fatigued.

E. WHAT TO SAY TO THE SUBJECT

Great care must be taken to prevent apprehension in the blindfolded subject and also to avoid giving any prejudicing cues as to the nature of the test. Moreover, the subject quite properly relies on the tester to place his hands in the precise and correct position on each occasion they are moved. A blindfolded subject should not be left in complete silence for more than a 15-second interval. The tester should repeat his remarks to the subject about concentrating on the size of blocks, and the like, during the period the subject is blindfolded. The words spoken by the tester to the subject are presented herewith in detail. These actual words should be typed out and kept by the tester to be read aloud until he is very well practiced. Do not paraphrase them unless it is essential for a particular subject's understanding.

Introduction

"We are doing some research on pain. There is evidence that the sense of touch is related to the way in which people experience pain and stress. This study does not involve subjecting you to pain or stress in any way. We are going to ask you some questions, and explore your sense of touch in these two fingers on each hand; that's all.

"There are no right or wrong answers. We are interested in the way in which *you* experience things; the only right answers are what *you* feel. Many people have done this before. It will take about an hour and a half.

"Let me explain what we are going to do. We'll place your right hand on a horizontal wooden block of a certain width; then, while you are still holding this block, we'll place your left hand on a horizontal block that tapers from a small width at the bottom to a greater width at the top. I will ask you to find a place on the tapered block that feels just as wide as the block in your right hand. Because the sense of touch is influenced by what you have been doing with your hands, you must rest these two fingers of both hands before we can use the blocks. Nothing should touch them while they rest. You can cross your arms or put them in any position so long as you keep your fingers from touching each other." The tester demonstrates the possible positions of arms and hands. He *must* watch the subject's fingers from now on. The subject now rests his hands for 45 minutes and during this time the tester should determine the handedness of the subject (see footnote 4), and collect other data that is required for the particular investigation. It is important *not* to leave the subject bored and unoccupied.

"I told you something about the blocks we are going to use. Well, we are ready for them now. Let me tell you what we'll do. We'll place your right hand on a horizontal block of a certain width, and your left on the longer block that tapers from a narrow width at the bottom to a wider width at the top. I'll ask you to find a spot on the tapered block that feels just as wide as the block in your right hand. We'll do this a few times and then place your

right hand on a different size block and ask you to rub it with thes
same two fingers. Remember, there are no right or wrong answer
—the only right answer is what you feel. Because it is essentia
that you judge by what you feel and not by what you see, we mus
cover your eyes. This part of the testing will take only a fev
minutes. While your eyes are covered I am going to have on thi
table only this stopwatch, this pad and pen, and the blocks.'
Make sure that the subject's chair is the proper distance from an(
facing the desk.

The tester now blindfolds the subject. "Does that seem comforta
ble? Can you see anything through the blindfold?" The tester the
places the tapered block and the measuring block, with stand
in the position for measuring. (See Fig. 29.)

"Let's put the two fingers of your right hand on a block; yo
can feel that the top slides and the block is the same width al
along. Now let's put your other two fingers on another block; yo
can feel again that the top slides, but this block gets wider an(
wider. Feel it." Encourage the subject to feel the tapered bloc
once, but do *not* allow him to go beyond the 8-inch mark, and se(
that his hand is returned to the bottom of the block.

"Now show me a spot on the tapered block which feels just a
wide as the block in your other hand. Find it as quickly *and a*
accurately *as you can. Say 'here,' when you have found it an(*
wait a moment *until I say 'all right'."* Tester records number o
tapered block. *"All right. Now, please return your hand to th(*
bottom of the tapered block and show me again a place on th(
tapered block which feels just as wide as the block in your othe
hand. Remember to say 'here,' and wait a moment until I sa
'all right'."

These instructions should be repeated a minimum of two times
subsequently when the tester feels *sure* that the subject knows th(
routine, he may say "now, show me again—again—and again,'
and so forth.

The tester records six measurements, being sure that the sub
ject's hand returns to the narrow end of the tapered block befor(
each measurement. To make recording possible the tester has t(
ask the subject to pause a moment when he has found the spot or
the tapered block that feels the same width. During the process o
measuring, the subject must never have his arms resting on th(
table. Immediately after the six measurements have been obtained,

the tester removes the subject's left hand from the tapered block.

"Now you may rest just this hand but be careful not to let the tips of your index finger or thumb touch each other or anything else."

The next words are spoken as the tester and the subject pick up the measuring block. The tester places the stimulating block on the stand, putting it in the proper position for stimulation, and then places the subject's hand on the block.

"Now we are going to pick up this right-hand block together. Hold it lightly here for a moment. Now we'll let go of this block, and put your fingers on a different block. When I say 'go ahead,' would you please rub this block along its length, back and forth, at whatever rate you like. I want you to concentrate on the width of the block, so I'm not going to talk to you about anything else until you finish rubbing."

The subject now begins the rubbing, and the tester sets the stopwatch. The subject should rest his arm on the table or a folded coat *during the period of rubbing only*. The tester should *frequently* say during this period, "Please concentrate on the width of the block" and "Just a few more seconds to go." After 90 seconds, the tester says:

"Now we are going to pick up this right-hand block together. Hold it lightly here for a moment. Now I am going to put these fingers onto another block; and I'll again put the fingers of your left hand on the tapered block."

The tester now returns the blocks and the subject's hands to the measuring position, repeats the instructions *italicized* on the previous page, and again records the four measurements. The process is repeated for another 90-second stimulation period and measurements, and then for a 120-second stimulation period and measurements. Blocks and recorded scores are then removed from the table and the blindfold from the subject.

"I'm just putting the blocks away. I'll be right with you. We're going to give your fingers a little rest, but don't touch anything with them. There will be no more rubbing. You will just give me four more measurements after this rest, and then we're all done."

After the 15 minutes of rest the blindfold is put on again and the four final measurements are made. Again the blocks and recorded scores must be put out of sight before the blindfold is finally removed from the subject.

F. SUMMARY

1. *Large Block*
   45 minutes of hand-resting
   Baseline . . . six measurements of 1½-inch block
   90-second stimulation   2½-inch block
   Four measurements   1½-inch block
   90-second stimulation   2½-inch block
   Four measurements   1½-inch block
   120-second stimulation   2½-inch block
   Four measurements   1½-inch block
   15 minutes of hand-resting
   Four measurements   1½-inch block

After a minimum of 48 hours interval

2. *Small Block*
   45 minutes of hand-resting
   Baseline . . . six measurements of 2-inch block
   90-second stimulation   1-inch block
   Four measurements   2-inch block
   90-second stimulation   1-inch block
   Four measurements   2-inch block
   120-second stimulation   1-inch block
   Four measurements   2-inch block
   15 minutes of hand-resting
   Four measurements   2-inch block [5]

[5] If lack of time makes the complete investigation described here unachievable then the following shortened forms are recommended:

   a. With normal adults, an approximation of the degree of reduction or augmentation can be obtained after three stimulation sessions, with only one sized-block—a ten minute procedure.

   b. With children and adolescents, the small- and large-block stimulation sessions are needed to determine the stimulus-governed trends, but the last quarter of an hour rest period and re-testing can be omitted on each occasion; thus two ten-minute procedures on separate days are involved.

   c. With neurological or psychiatric patients, it is urged that the full procedure be used; two half-hour testing sessions on separate days are involved.

   DO NOT OMIT THE 45 MINUTE HAND-RESTING PERIOD WITH ANY GROUP. THE RESULTS WILL BE AFFECTED IN AN UNPREDICTABLE MANNER DEPENDING ON WHAT EACH PERSON HAPPENED TO HAVE BEEN DOING PRIOR TO

G. COMPLETING A RECORD

Here are examples of a recording of results (see Table 17 *et seq.*).[6] Only the last four measurements of the baseline are used. The first two are practice measurements and are necessary to enable the blindfolded subject to become familiar with the feel of the apparatus and with the procedure. An average is taken of each group of four measurements (see Table 20). The baseline average (labeled I in Table 20) is subtracted from each average to give the three differences which occurred after stimulation (the lines labeled II, III, and IV). Averaging them gives the final average which, when compared with the comparable average for the small-block stimulation, gives rise to a classification of the subject as a reducer, augmenter, moderate, or stimulus-governed. In many investigations the concern, however, will be with the degree of reduction and augmentation rather than with an absolute classification.

When this final average indicates that the subject has reduced by 1.8 inches or more—on stimulation with either the large block or the small block—he is classified as a reducer (see Table 20). When the final average indicates that the subject has augmented by 1.8 inches or more, he is classified as an augmenter (see Table 21). (As the baseline value is subtracted from each set of measurements after stimulation, it becomes apparent that reducing is indicated by a [−] average and augmenting by a [+] average.) When neither average reaches −1.8 inches or +1.8 inches, the subject is classified as a moderate (see Tables 22 and 23).

When the average reaches or exceeds −1.8 inches on the large-block stimulation session and +1.8 inches on the small block stimulation session—that is to say, the score of a reducer *and* an augmenter are present in the *same* person—the subject is classified

---

TESTING, AND THE DEGREE OF REDUCTION AND AUGMENTATION ALREADY INDUCED IN HIM BY SUCH ACTIVITY. THE AMOUNT OF ADDITIONAL REDUCTION OR AUGMENTATION THAT CAN STILL BE DEMONSTRATED IS THEN MISLEADING AS TO THE CHARACTERISTIC PERCEPTUAL MODULATION OF EACH PERSON.

[6] These actual records have been chosen because they present a particularly wide range of scores.

TABLE 20

COMPLETED RECORD OF A REDUCER (INCLUDING COMPUTATIONS)
(LARGE-BLOCK STIMULATION)

Series of Measurements	Practice Trials		(1)	(2)	(3)	(4)	Total	Average	Difference from Baseline Average
I (Baseline)	(11 7/8)	(12 3/8)	14 2/8	14 4/8	14 2/8	14 6/8	57.75	14.43	
II (After 90-second stimulation)			12 6/8	13 2/8	13 4/8	14	53.5	13.37	−1.06
III (After 180-second stimulation)			11	13 2/8	12 3/8	12 7/8	49.5	12.37	−2.06
IV (After 300-second stimulation)			9 2/8	10 4/8	11 4/8	12 4/8	43.75	10.94	−3.49
Rest Period									
V (After 15-minute rest period)			10 3/8	11	11 3/8	12 1/8	44.875	11.22	−3.21

Final Average Modulation $= \frac{-6.61}{3} = -2.20$

TABLE 21

COMPLETED RECORD OF AN AUGMENTER (INCLUDING COMPUTATIONS)
(SMALL-BLOCK STIMULATION)

Series of Measurements	Practice Trials		(1)	(2)	(3)	(4)	Total	Average	Difference from Baseline Average
I (Baseline)	(10 7/8)	(11 7/8)	10 7/8	10 7/8	11 2/8	11 1/8	44.125	11.03	
II (After 90-second stimulation)			13 3/8	13 4/8	12 3/8	12 3/8	51.625	12.91	+1.88
III (After 180-second stimulation)			13 6/8	13 3/8	13 2/8	13	53.375	13.34	+2.31
IV (After 300-second stimulation)			14 6/8	12 6/8	13 6/8	14 1/8	55.375	13.84	+2.81
Rest Period									
V (After 15-minute rest period)			14 3/8	14 6/8	14 3/8	15	58.5	14.63	+3.60

Final Average Modulation $= \frac{7}{3} = +2.33$

TABLE 22

COMPLETED RECORD OF A MODERATE (INCLUDING COMPUTATIONS)
(LARGE-BLOCK STIMULATION)

Series of Measurements	Practice Trials		(1)	(2)	(3)	(4)	Total	Average	Difference from Baseline Average
I (Baseline)	(9⁴⁄₈)	(8⁴⁄₈)	8⁴⁄₈	8	9¹⁄₈	9	34.625	8.66	
II (After 90-second stimulation)			9²⁄₈	8⁴⁄₈	7⁴⁄₈	6⁵⁄₈	31.875	7.97	−.69
III (After 180-second stimulation)			9⁶⁄₈	8⁷⁄₈	8	8¹⁄₈	34.75	8.69	+.03
IV (After 300-second stimulation)			8³⁄₈	8	9	9	34.625	8.59	−.07
Rest Period									
V (After 15-minute rest period)			7⁶⁄₈	8³⁄₈	8²⁄₈	8⁷⁄₈	33.25	8.31	−.35

Final Average Modulation $= \frac{-.73}{3} = -.24$

TABLE 23
Completed Record of a Moderate (Including Computations) (Small-Block Stimulation)

Series of Measurements	Practice Trials		(1)	(2)	(3)	(4)	Total	Average	Difference from Baseline Average
I (Baseline)	(17 1/8)	(17 4/8)	16 6/8	16 7/8	16 5/8	17 6/8	68.0	17	
II (After 90-second stimulation)			17 6/8	18	17 4/8	17 1/8	70.375	17.59	+.59
III (After 180-second stimulation)			17 4/8	18 3/8	18	17 7/8	71.75	17.94	+.94
IV (After 300-second stimulation)			17	17 6/8	18	18 1/8	70.75	17.69	+.69
Rest Period									
V (After 15-minute rest period)			17 2/8	16 4/8	16 2/8	17 5/8	67.625	16.91	−.09

Final Average Modulation $= \frac{2.22}{3} = +.74$

as stimulus-governed (as when Tables 20 and 21 represent the scores of a single subject).[7]

Thus an augmenter needs to have an average increase of 1.8 inches or more on one of the stimulation sessions and three possibilities exist for the average from the other session; (1) It could also show an increase of 1.8 inches or more. (2) It could show an increase of less than 1.8 inches—that is, fall within the moderate range. (3) It might show a decrease of less than 1.8 inches, again falling within the moderate range.

On the other hand, a reducer needs to have an average decrease of 1.8 inches or more on one of the stimulation sessions and three possibilities exist for the average from the other session: (1) It could also show a decrease of 1.8 inches or more. (2) It could show a decrease of less than 1.8 inches and fall within the moderate range. (3) It might show an increase of less than 1.8 inches, again falling within the moderate range.

The tester needs to check that both sessions were carried out at the same time of day, when the subject was not fatigued, sick, or had taken any drugs; that the enviromental conditions were constant and the same tester completed both sessions; that there was no excessive stimulation during either session, from bright lights, a loud noise, and so on; that the subject was not under emotional pressures during either session and that as far as can be ascertained his subjective state was comparable on the two occasions; and, finally, that in females testing was not carried out in the premenstrual days and that both sessions had been completed during the same time in the menstrual cycle.

Such checking is always important but it is essential when the third possibility listed above occurs, that is, when one of the sessions provides high moderate scores with a different sign from the other. Moreover, double checking should *never* be omitted when stimulus-governed scores are found.

[7] A negatively stimulus-governed person is a rarity, that is, someone whose average score is at least +1.8 inches on the large-block stimulation session and at least −1.8 inches on the small-block stimulation session.

A word of warning is proper here. You will see that it would occasionally be possible to obtain a pseudo-stimulus-governed score. For example, if prior to the testing with the large stimulus the patient had been subjected to a drug or to one of the other means by which an augmenter can be changed into a reducer, we would obtain an "induced" reducer score; but, if he were tested without any such interference with the small block, he would give us an augmenter score.

It is clear that as in a normal adult population there is a significant positive correlation between scores obtained during the two sessions, a large deviation in an adult is suspect. These stimulus-governed trends occur, however, in children and to a lesser extent among adolescents; they are present during premenstrual days in females and in periods of fatigue and sickness in any subject.

The figures so far have all referred to linear measurements read off from the ruler attached to the tapered block marked in inches and eighths of an inch. These are, of course, not equivalent to the amount of reduction or augmentation of the width of the measuring block but are proportional to it. With the standardized apparatus we are using in the Boston area, conversion to the equivalent width expressed in millimeters, from the linear measurement of the tapered block, can be achieved by multiplying the linear measurement by three. The findings and the categories reported are based on results obtained with these standardized techniques and apparatus, on many hundreds of subjects.

In spite of our best endeavors to make this text of instruction as comprehensive as possible, we have found that after an investigator has absorbed all that this description can teach him, in order to avoid errors he needs to be supervised for at least one session by someone who is completely conversant with these techniques.

Appendix B

Weights

Comparison of Augmentation and Reduction in the Kinesthetic Perception of Size and the Perception of Weight

The experiment in which the perception of weight was compared with the standard kinesthetic method of measuring perceptual reactance required somewhat different techniques. It is therefore described separately and in some detail in this appendix.

This investigation was carried out on male juvenile delinquents. The positive correlation between the measurements of size and weight is reported in the "Modalities" section of chapter 1.

Subjects. Twenty-two male adolescent delinquent subjects were tested. Sixteen were reducers, augmenters, or moderates; six were stimulus-governed.

Apparatus. A set of 25 uniform, blackened plastic containers, measuring 1½ inches x 2 inches x 5¾ inches (a size that can be easily held in the average adult hand) were used as weights. They ranged from 1 to 25 ounces by 1 ounce increments.

The experiment was comparable in design to the one on kinesthetic size as described in Appendix A. As in the experiments on size, different sets of stimulating and measuring weights were used for large-weight and small-weight stimulation in order to avoid excessive practice with weights of exactly the same amount. Thus *measuring* and *stimulating* weights were added to the regular series.

For large-weight stimulation:
For measuring   9 oz.
For stimulation   18 oz.

For small-weight stimulation:
For measuring   15 oz.
For stimulation   6 oz.

Different proportions with which I have experimented were too heavy to be manipulated in the required amount of time or appeared to present too small a contrast effect.[1]

Procedure. The sessions for large and small weights were scheduled in random order at the same time of day, with an interval of at least 48 hours between the two.

Each session commenced with a resting period for the hands. After the experimental procedure had been explained to the subject, he was blindfolded. The measuring weight was then placed in his right hand with his palm facing upwards. Into his left hand, also with the palm facing upwards, were placed consecutively each of the series of weights, commencing with the lightest weight. This procedure was continued until the subject felt that the weight in his left hand equaled the one in his right hand. (He was permitted to request that the weights be decreased as well as increased until he found the weight that seemed to him equivalent.) The number of the weight chosen was then recorded. The subject completed two such estimates of equivalence.

His left hand was then rested on the table while into his right hand was placed the stimulating weight. He was asked to attend to the weight his hand was supporting, and to lift his hand upwards and downwards, at a constant rate, with the palm facing upwards, until told to stop.

There were three stimulation sessions, lasting respectively 90 seconds, 90 seconds, and 120 seconds. After each of these sessions the subject made two measures of equivalence of the measuring weight held in his right hand with the series of weights placed in his left hand.

Statistical Analysis. The perceptual reactance shown with *weights,* based on scores from both the small-block and large-block stimulation, were averaged for each subject. A parallel statistical analysis

---

[1] In addition to the weight values listed, the following alternative weights have been tried: *For large-weight stimulation*—measuring weight 9 ounces, stimulating weight 15 ounces. *For small-weight stimulation*—measuring weight 12 ounces, stimulating weight 6 ounces.

was made for the corresponding investigation of kinesthetic augmentation and reduction in the *perception of size* by the same subjects. For the 16 reducers, augmenters, and moderates, a product-moment correlation was found between weight and size augmentation and reduction. It was $r = .53$. The statistical significance of the value indicates a positive association between the two perceptual differences being explored.

In addition, the six stimulus-governed delinquents, identified by their behavior on the "size" tests, were given both the large-weight and small-weight stimulations. The measure of the extent of their stimulus-governed tendencies was compared with the spread between those same scores in the other 16 delinquents, who were reducers, augmenters, and moderates. The figures were 2.13 ounces and 1.10 ounces respectively. This spread for the stimulus-governed was significantly greater, as shown by a Mann-Whitney U-test (one-tail, .05 probability).

The findings in the perception of weight add to the accumulating evidence that what is being measured kinesthetically is one aspect of the generalized tendency for the reducer to diminish the perception of stimulation and for the augmenter to enlarge it—two contrasting processes manifesting themselves in persons with differing characteristics.

Appendix C

Some Further Correlations Related to Reliability

Correlation of Change in Estimated Size after 180 Seconds with That after a Further 120 Seconds

It was reported in chapter 1 that the split-half reliability correlation coefficients of the kinesthetic method for measuring perceptual reactance were found to be .979 for a group of 25 school children and .973 for a group of 33 student nurses. In addition, the amount of change after 180 seconds of stimulation with the large block has been correlated with that obtained after a further 120 seconds of stimulation in three groups studied by us. The correlation coefficients are:

A. With 23 subjects, members of the staff at the
   Boston Sanatorium $r = .89$
B. With 22 patients and some members of the hos-
   pital staff *not* used in other studies $r = .90$
C. With 23 dental outpatients $r = .86$[1]

[1] Reliability figures, using large-block stimulation alone, are reported by Eysenck (1955); in a group of 14 hysterics the values were .78 and .86 and, in a group of 14 dysthymics, .93 and .94. Other colleagues, in personal communications, tell of studies yielding similar values.

A repeat-reliability study, using comparable apparatus (large-block stimulation) with 154 college sophomores, was reported by Spitz and Lipman (1960) to yield a correlation of .74. (The latter figures are undoubtedly attenuated in that, for example, the kinesthetic testing was not preceded by an adequate rest period that would insure the subjects not being in a state of augmentation or reduction while they were being investigated.)

The Correlation between Large- and Small-Block Stimulation in Adolescents

It was reported in chapter 1 that in a group of adults (age range, 23 to 57; average age, 35.5 years), the correlation between small- and large-block stimulation is .72. It is to be expected that in a group containing more adolescents and children the correlation would be lower, since stimulus-governed tendencies, that reduce this correlation, diminish with increasing maturity (see chapter 5).

In a study of an adolescent group of 13 female Wellesley College students (age range, 17 to 21; average age, 19) who were given both large- and small-block stimulation with a minimum of 48 hours intervening, the correlation of the average change after large-block stimulation with that after small-block stimulation was .60 (significant of a positive relationship between the two at a $p = .025$, one-tail test). The frequency distributions of this group are presented in Tables 24 and 25.

In a still younger group of 58 public school children and student nurses in the Boston area, described in chapter 5 (age range, 14 to 26, average age, 18) the correlation of the average change after large-block stimulation with that after small-block stimulation was .40, significant of a positive relationship between the two at a probability of .005, one-tail test. The frequency distributions of this group are presented in Tables 26 and 27.[2]

As the stimulus-governed tendencies of a young child are increasingly inhibited with maturity, one can recognize the characteristic augmenter not only by his augmenting scores on small-block stimulation, but in his inhibition of reduction on the large-block stimulation. The characteristic reducer in contrast, is recognized not only by the reduction he shows on large-block stimulation, but by his inhibition of augmentation on small-block stimulation.

The degree of such inhibition does not appear to be proportional to the amount of reduction or augmentation displayed when one looks at one-half of the picture on its own. It seems to express a personal characteristic of that particular augmenter or reducer.

---

[2] As the work has progressed we have learned to control an increasing number of variables that alter perceptual reactance. At the time of the schoolchildren's study we were not yet aware of the alterations associated with some of these variables, and it is possible that this ignorance has contributed, to some extent, to the lower correlation between large- and small-block stimulation in comparison with the adult group.

TABLE 24

FREQUENCY DISTRIBUTION OF LARGE-BLOCK STIMULATION
SCORES FOR WELLESLEY STUDENTS

Change in Subjective Size of Block (mm)	Number of Subjects
+9.00 or more	0
+7.20 to +8.99	0
+5.40 to +7.19	0
+3.60 to +5.39	0
+1.80 to +3.59	0
0.00 to +1.79	0
−1.79 to 0.00	1
−3.59 to −1.80	5
−5.39 to −3.60	3
−7.19 to −5.40	3
−9.00 or less	1

N (female) = 13;   age range = 17 to 21;   average age = 19.

TABLE 25

FREQUENCY DISTRIBUTION OF SMALL-BLOCK STIMULATION
SCORES FOR WELLESLEY STUDENTS

Change in Subjective Size of Block (mm)	Number of Subjects
+9.00 or more	1
+7.20 to +8.99	0
+5.40 to +7.19	2
+3.60 to +5.39	1
+1.80 to +3.59	6
0.00 to +1.79	1
−1.79 to 0.00	2
−3.59 to −1.80	0
−5.39 to −3.60	0
−7.19 to −5.40	0
−8.99 to −7.20	0
−9.00 or less	0

N (female) = 13;   age range = 17 to 21;   average age = 19.

Obviously, a person's experience consists of both types of contrast effects and his perceptual behavior under both conditions concerns us. It is, therefore, most desirable, whenever possible, to determine perceptual reactance by using scores from both large- and small-block stimulation. The need for such a "bifocal" picture has become increasingly clear with accumulating data.

The conditions of clinical research often limit the number of times a patient can be seen. In these experiments we were often forced to use large- or small-block stimulation alone, to estimate,

TABLE 26

FREQUENCY DISTRIBUTION OF LARGE-BLOCK STIMULATION
SCORES FOR A GROUP OF SCHOOL CHILDREN
AND NURSING STUDENTS

Change in Estimated Size (mm)	Number of Persons
+9.00 or more	1
+7.20 to +8.99	0
+5.40 to +7.19	1
+3.60 to +5.39	1
+1.80 to +3.59	3
0.00 to +1.79	9
−1.79 to 0.00	12
−3.59 to −1.80	12
−5.39 to −3.60	14
−7.19 to −5.40	2
−8.99 to −7.20	1
−9.00 or less	2

$N = 58$;   age range = 14 to 26;   average age = 18.

TABLE 27

FREQUENCY DISTRIBUTION OF SMALL-BLOCK STIMULATION
SCORES FOR A GROUP OF SCHOOL CHILDREN
AND NURSING STUDENTS

Change in Estimated Size (mm)	Number of Persons
+9.00 or more	6
+7.20 to +8.99	7
+5.40 to +7.19	6
+3.60 to +5.39	6
+1.80 to +3.59	8
0.00 to +1.80	5
−1.79 to 0.00	8
−3.59 to −1.80	7
−5.39 to −3.60	1
−7.19 to −5.40	2
−8.99 to −7.20	0
−9.00 or less	2

$N = 58$;   age range = 14 to 26;   average age = 18.

for example, the effect of a pain-relieving procedure. The positive correlation between large-block stimulation and small indicates that, in using only one contrasted size, we are actually underrating the existing perceptual differences between the augmenter and reducer.

Appendix D

Baseline Scores

The effect of stimulation on the perception of the reducer is to make him perceive *what he is holding in the hand used for stimulation* as being decreased in size. We have been making our investigations by stimulating the dominant hand—the right hand in right-handed people—and having the measures of equivalence made on the tapered block with the left hand. Thus underlying all the findings on kinesthetic perceptual reactance is that the right hand should be stimulated (so that, for example, in a reducer its perception of size is reduced), whereas the left hand should be kept as unstimulated as is possible so that its perception of size remains relatively unchanged. As a result, a comparison of the unstimulated left hand with the right hand demonstrates the reduction taking place for the right hand.

Nevertheless, before any deliberate stimulation of the right hand is begun, the left hand, in sliding up and down the tapered block to find the equivalent width, is being inadvertently stimulated. This inadvertent stimulation of the left hand should, for the *reducer,* result in his perception of the size of the *tapered block* being reduced. That is to say, the reducer would tend to find the portion of the tapered block he is holding narrower than it had seemed to him before the inadvertent stimulation, and he would therefore try to find a *wider* bit of the tapered block to equate with the measuring block of constant size held in his right hand. For that reason we would expect the reducer's left hand to be affected by his original contacts with the tapered block, so that he would demonstrate the reduction taking place for it by choosing *larger* widths of this block as his equivalence judgment.[1]

In contrast, we would expect the augmenter to perceive the portion of the tapered block he is holding as being wider than it had been before the inadvertent stimulation of the left hand, so that he would choose a narrower portion of the tapered block as equivalent to the measuring block held in his right hand. Thus we would expect that, even after the small amount of stimulation with the tapered block on the left hand involved in making the original equivalence judgments (approximately 60 seconds in all), the reducer would differ from the augmenter because the former is diminishing the size while the latter is enlarging it. The reducer would therefore choose larger widths while the augmenter would choose narrower widths with his left hand. This is exactly what we found (see Table 28).[2]

Indeed, with certain important exceptions one can *start* identifying the reducer from the larger baseline measurements that he provides.

The stimulation sustained by the left hand on the tapered block, while obtaining the two sets of 12 measurements, causes the augmenter to give us smaller scores and the reducer larger scores. This attenuates the differences in reduction and augmentation obtained after the deliberate stimulation of the right hand on the measuring block, for these latter effects are dependent on the *difference* in the degree of stimulation sustained by the two hands.

The initial effect of stimulation in inducing reduction or augmentation is particularly pronounced; that is to say, the second period of stimulation, although of equal length, does not cause as pronounced alteration in perceived size as does the first period (see

[1] In one experiment, the usual technique was altered so that the hand on the tapered block was stimulated by rubbing a larger block, and the hand on the measuring block was left free of any stimulation. Here the hypothesis was that, when the subject is a reducer, that particular part of the tapered block that was judged as equivalent in width would have been reduced subjectively, so that it seemed smaller. The reducer, therefore, would move to a *larger* width to find equivalence. (This larger width would also have been subjectively reduced and now would appear to be of the size equivalent to the block in the other hand.) Thus, as the hand on the tapered block reduces, it chooses larger widths equivalent to the block held in the other hand. The results of the experiment supported this hypothesis.

[2] The presence of a number of extreme reducers among the delinquents contributed to the pronounced differences between reducers and augmenters in this group.

TABLE 28

COMPARISON BETWEEN REDUCERS AND AUGMENTERS ON BASELINE SCORES

NAME OF GROUP	MEAN BASELINE SCORE ON LARGE-BLOCK TEST (mm)			MEAN BASELINE SCORE ON SMALL-BLOCK TEST (mm)		
	Re-ducers	Aug-menters	Standard Error of Difference between Means	Re-ducers	Aug-menters	Standard Error of Difference between Means
Cambridge school children	31.59 (N = 5)	26.97 (N = 9)	3.42	40.47 (N = 5)	36.06 (N = 9)	2.34
Student nurses	28.77 (N = 4)	27.00 (N = 10)	2.25	41.79 (N = 4)	36.30 (N = 10)	1.53
Delinquents [a]	32.34 (N = 19)	26.52** (N = 8)	2.25	39.06 (N = 19)	33.42* (N = 8)	2.52

Note: The categories Reducer and Augmenter are based on both the large- and the small-block scores.
* The difference is significant at the .025 level for a one-tail test.
** The difference is significant at the .01 level for a one-tail test.
[a] Delinquent group tested in 1960.

Table 29).[3] It follows that the initial contact of the left hand with the tapered block during the baseline measurements is the most potent period for inducing the augmentation or reduction in that hand.

Being conscious of this problem, inherent in the use of the tapered block, we have tried various alternatives. For example, for a while we used fingerprints in a plate of salt instead of the tapered block to obtain the equivalent width of the blocks held in the right hand, and observed pronounced reducing and augmenting in this manner. Subsequently, we inked the fingers to make prints on paper, a method which gave us permanent records. Although clear evidence of augmenting and reducing was demonstrated (see Fig. 8 in chapter 1), the precise and consistent measurements provided by the use of the tapered block were lacking. It appears that the

[3] In addition, during the first period of stimulation, the reduction induced for the right hand equals and then outstrips that occasioned for the left hand through the inadvertent stimulation by the tapered block. Thus the scores for perceptual reactance understate the total effect of the initial stimulation.

TABLE 29

NAME OF GROUP	Difference between baseline scores of reducers and augmenters (mm)	Difference between scores of reducers and augmenters after 90 seconds of stimulation (mm)	Difference between scores of reducers and augmenters after 180 seconds of stimulation (mm)	Difference between scores of reducers and augmenters after 300 seconds of stimulation (mm)
	Differences with Large-Block Test			
Cambridge school children: reducers ($N = 5$) augmenters ($N = 9$)	4.62	−3.24	−9.87	−10.32
Student nurses: reducers ($N = 4$) augmenters ($N = 10$)	1.77	−4.86	−2.82	−5.22
	Differences with Small-Block Test			
Cambridge school children: reducers ($N = 5$) augmenters ($N = 9$)	4.41	−11.34	−10.95	−11.79
Student nurses: reducers ($N = 4$) augmenters ($N = 10$)	5.49	−13.02	−16.47	−13.20
Delinquents: reducers ($N = 19$) augmenters ($N = 8$)	5.64	−5.94	−8.28	−8.61

chief defect in these alternatives that attempted to dispense with
the tapered block was that the subject was not holding between the
fingers of his left hand anything comparable to the measuring block
held between the fingers of his right hand. To get a precise measure of subjective equivalence the experiences for the two hands
need to be as nearly identical as possible. Moreover, people can
measure more accurately an object held between the fingers than
an empty space between the fingers. So it turns out that the tapered
block provides the more reliable and consistent measurements,

provided always that one understands about the inadvertent stimulation that this block causes to the left hand.

Moreover, if the tendency to reduction is increased by the
administration of alcohol to an augmenter for example, the hand
on the tapered block is going to be more susceptible to the unin-
tentional reduction caused by the movement up and down and will
choose an even larger portion of the tapered block than previously.
The baseline scores with alcohol show precisely this effect.

In fact, as will be seen in Table 30 for alcohol, aspirin, and

TABLE 30

CHANGE IN BASELINE SCORES OF AUGMENTERS
UNDER EXPERIMENTAL CONDITIONS

EXPERIMENTAL CONDITION	MEAN BASELINE SCORE OF AUGMENTERS ON LARGE-BLOCK TEST (mm)	
	Neutral Condition	Experimental Condition
Alcohol	23.04 (N = 9)	31.05* (N = 9)
Aspirin	25.86 (N = 10)	35.34* (N = 10)
Stimulation with sound	24.75 (N = 9)	31.32* (N = 9)

Note: The Wilcoxen Matched-Pairs Sign-Ranks test was
used with the above data.
* The difference is significant at the .005 level for a one-
tail test.

audio-analgesia—all three of which cause increased reduction—
the baseline scores for the augmenters change and become larger.
These three pain relieving methods did not cause a significant
change in the baseline scores of reducers. As reported in chapters
3 and 4, reducers showed no significant change in perceptual modulation in these three studies. What this means is that the effect of
stimulation by the tapered block on the augmenter, under the influence of these conditions that increase reduction, is to cause his
left hand—as well as his right hand—to demonstrate the increased
reduction.

As was explained above, the higher scores of the reducer as

compared with the augmenter in the baseline scores was dependent on the inadvertent rubbing of the tapered block for approximately 60 seconds. The differences between the reducer and augmenter on subsequent scores are generally greater after 300 seconds of deliberate stimulation than after 90 seconds of stimulation. We would therefore expect that the difference between them at 300 seconds should exceed the difference on the baseline. That this is so is shown in Table 29.

It thus appears that a considerable variety of predictions about the baseline are borne out—predictions that were made on the assumption that in the baseline scores we are witnessing the effect of the unavoidable stimulation of the tapered block on the left hand.

Appendix E

Neurophysiological Studies of Reduction and Augmentation

By M. S. Buchsbaum

Individual Differences and Evoked Potentials

Like the silhouette of a face, the evoked potential curve shows a tremendous variety of differences in individuals. These differences concern not just waveform or amplitude but also the changes in evoked potentials caused by experimental tasks or pharmacological treatment. Conventional neurophysiology initially tended to minimize the value of scalp evoked potentials and to attribute the variation to artifacts or to poor control of stimulus delivery. For researchers involved in perceptual and cognitive style or personality, however, the news that people are really different came as no shock. Evoked potential technique seemed a way to separate attention, motivation, and various performance variables by examining each evoked potential component in succession. Differences between individuals in the way evoked potentials change with increasing stimulus intensity appear especially striking (Fig. 34). Most typically, visual evoked potentials in subjects responding to light flashes increase in amplitude with increasing stimulus intensity up to an intermediate intensity and then level off or decrease; individual differences are quite prominent (Rietveld 1963; Rietveld and Tordoir 1965; Armington 1964*a*, 1964*b*; Shagass et al. 1965; Vaughan and Hull 1965; Shipley et al. 1966; Buchsbaum and Silverman 1968).

Decreases in amplitude with increasing intensity appear at least partly to represent central inhibitory processes, rather than peripheral adjustment mechanisms. The high intensity stimulus does

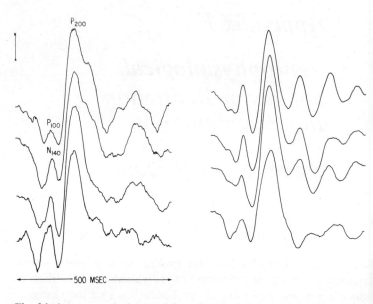

Fig. 34. Average evoked potentials to four intensities of light flash: top to bottom, dim to bright. The individual on the left shows augmenting—increasing amplitude with increasing stimulus intensity for component P1 (P100)–N1 (N140). The individual on the right shows reducing—decreasing amplitude with increasing stimulus intensity for P1–N1 (Buchsbaum and Pfefferbaum 1971).

indeed appear to get into the central nervous system in reducers; simultaneous electroretinographic and vertex evoked potential recordings show almost linear amplitude/intensity relationships at the retina but reducing for later vertex components (Armington 1964*a*, 1964*b*). Further, evoked potential latency seems to decrease fairly linearly with increasing intensity in the same subjects who show reducing in amplitude (DeVoe et al. 1968). Other authors have also noted this latency vs. amplitude difference (Wooten 1972; Clynes et al. 1964; Vaughan and Hull 1965). Within the central nervous system, we have found reducing more prominent at vertex than over occipital leads, and more prominent for P100 than for P200 (Buchsbaum and Pfefferbaum 1971), also suggesting central inhibition rather than peripheral adjustment.

We have devoted some attention to the problem of relationship between pupillary diameter and visual evoked potential amplitude/

ntensity slopes. Data from our laboratory and elsewhere do not
upport a relationship between late evoked potential components
ecorded from vertex and pupillary diameter. Two naturalistic
tudies (Kooi and Bagchi 1964, and Richey et al. 1966) failed to
onfirm any pupil–evoked potential correlation for the vertex lead.
est-retest reliabilities for evoked potential amplitude/intensity
lopes were not decreased by stabilizing pupillary diameter with
ilocarpine (Soskis and Shagass 1974). In a study on eight normal
olunteers in our laboratory (Buchsbaum, forthcoming) no signifi-
ant vertex visual evoked potential effects were seen in subjects with
upils either dilated with neosynephrine or constricted with pilo-
arpine.

Reducing in the auditory system has been widely noted (see
Buchsbaum 1976 for review) and possible central inhibitory mecha-
isms are discussed by Picton (1970) and Atkinson (1976). Simi-
arly, somatosensory evoked potentials show non-monotonic
unctions (see Buchsbaum 1976).

Comparison Between Reduction and Augmentation in the Kinesthetic Perception of Size and Evoked Potential

The relationship between evoked potential measurements of aug-
nentation and reduction and the perceptual approach[1] can be tested
n two ways: first by correlations between the two measures of
timulus response style obtained from the same individuals and
econd by finding the postulated correlates of perceptual reactance
n augmenters and reducers selected by the evoked potential
neasurements.

Following the first technique, Buchsbaum and Silverman re-
orted a significant correlation between the evoked potential aug-
nenting/reducing measure and scores on Silverman's modification
f the perceptual approach procedure. Blacker et al. (1968), using
ight flashes, and Spilker and Callaway (1969b), using sine-wave
nodulated light, also reported a significant correlation. Borge
1973) also noted evoked potential reducers to be reducers on the
perceptual approach, but used a different evoked potential measure.

Buchsbaum and Pfefferbaum (1971) located a group of 10

[1]The term "perceptual approach" is used throughout Appendix E to
indicate reduction and augmentation as measured by the kinesthetic
perception of size.

extreme augmenters and 10 extreme reducers using the evoke
potential procedure by testing 66 normal male college students. Th
center group and those individuals without clearly identifiabl
P100–N140 peaks were excluded. Extreme reducers on the evoke
potential (as defined by decreases in P100–N140 amplitude wit
increasing intensity) had significantly greater reducing scores on th
large-block part of the perceptual approach than did the evoke
potential augmenters (reported in Schooler et al. 1976). Schooler e
al. (1976) also reported a significant correlation between vertex P10
amplitude/intensity slope and the large-block plus small-bloc
perceptual approach score ($r = .41$) in a population of 40 hospitalize
schizophrenics. Barnes (1976) reviews relationships between evoke
potential and perceptual reactance.

Genetic Factors

Evoked potential waveforms have been widely reported to sho
strong genetic influences (e.g. Dustman and Beck 1965; Lewis et al
1972; and Rust 1975). The evoked potential augmenting/reducin
measure has been studied in 33 pairs of monozygotic and 34 pairs o
dizygotic twins (Fig. 35; Buchsbaum 1974). Significantly highe
intraclass correlations were found in the monozygotic pairs than i
the dizygotic pairs for three measures of the P100 amplitude/inten
sity slope, P100–N140 peak-to-trough amplitude, the 76–112 mse
mean deviation measure, and the amplitude for a single coordinate o
exactly 100 msec (Buchsbaum 1974). These significant finding
arose largely from the monozygotic twin pair similarities (intraclas
$r = .54$ to .68); dizygotic intraclass correlations were often nea
zero. If the monozygotic correlation is more than twice the dizygoti
correlation, simple additive genic variance does not account for th
heritability. The implication is that several loci and/or dominance
epistasis, or dominance interactions may be involved.

   In data collected on the families of normal controls and o
psychiatric patients with affective disorders, significant intraclass
correlations were noted in offspring-offspring (intraclass $r = .30$
and sibling-sibling (.29) comparisons—both were higher than the
correlation observed in the dizygotic twin pairs (Gershon and
Buchsbaum 1977). However, since the amplitude/intensity slope
was significantly elevated in the patients with affective illness and in
their relatives, the increased variance due to sampling from the

TWIN PAIR I   TWIN PAIR 2

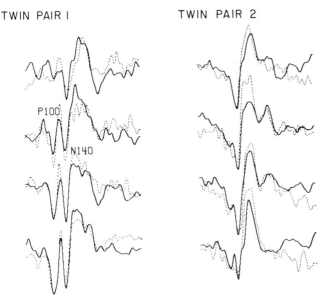

Fig. 35. Visual evoked potentials in two pairs of Mz twins. Illustrated are evoked potentials to four intensities of light, as in Fig. 34. For each pair, the evoked potential is shown as a solid line for one twin and as a dotted line for the co-twin. Note similarity in latency of peaks, waveform, and changes with stimulus intensity. For Pair 1, component P100–N140 increases markedly with stimulus intensity (augmenting), and for Pair 2, the component decreases with stimulus intensity (reducing) (Buchsbaum 1974).

extremes of the population distribution may explain the higher correlations.

It was also of interest that individuals in this sample tended to marry individuals with similar perceptual style; significant intraclass correlations were found between evoked potential amplitude/intensity slopes for husbands and wives.

Recording Evoked Potential Augmenting/Reducing

In our initial studies, evoked potential augmenting/reducing was measured with Grass-photostimulator flashes (10 microsecond duration) delivered to the subjects' closed eyelids at a distance of 100 cm. This procedure tended to minimize eye movement, but presented several problems: individual differences in eyelid pigmentation might affect evoked potential amplitude, closed eyes promoted drowsiness, and randomization of flash intensity was technically difficult to achieve. We were also concerned that flash stimuli might involve both "on" and "off" responses superimposed which might well have different amplitude/intensity gradients. Currently we use a 17" x 22" translucent plastic screen rear-illuminated by fluorescent tubes (driven by a Silconix unit) 50 cm from the subject with open eyes. This light source can be turned on in 3 msec and remain on for 500 msec so that only "on" responses to the light are evoked. On-line computer control (Coppola 1977) allows complete randomization of flash intensity over a fifteen-fold range from 2 to 250 foot-lamberts. This intensity range is extended by adding a second set of fluorescent tubes covered with 10% or 1% transmission neutral density filters.

EEG is recorded vertex to right ear with left ear ground and low pass filtered at 40 Hz since we are primarily interested in the P100–N140–P200 complex. Averages of 64 presentations of each stimulus intensity are usually adequate for these visual stimuli.

Measurement of the Evoked Potential Waveform

The measurement of evoked potential amplitude is complicated by the great individual variation in component waveform. While initially most investigators attempted to identify specific peaks, numerical area measures and factor analytic approaches are now becoming more common. As a measure of perceptual style, we needed an amplitude/intensity measure that was stable over repeated testing in the same individual; high heritability was also a useful criterion for certain familial studies of psychiatric patients. We tested our sample of 34 adult monozygotic twins twice, two or more weeks apart, which provided an opportunity to compare various evoked potential measurements. Evoked potentials to four intensities of light (Silconix photostimulator and random sequence delivery [Buchsbaum 1974]) were available with a prestimulus baseline. In these evoked potentials, P100 and N140 were visually identified for each of the four intensities for each session on each twin. The amplitude/intensity slope was calculated using least square regression for the four amplitudes measured peak-to-trough as well as prestimulus baseline to P100 peak. In addition, the area under the curve between 76 and 112 msec was calculated in several different ways (mean

bsolute deviation, mean signed deviation, root-mean-square devia-
ion, all relative to the mean of the evoked potential or prestimulus
baseline). The area time limits were based on the distribution of
atency for P100 as visually identified.

The measure with the highest test-retest ($r = .63$, $p < .001$) was
he mean absolute deviation calculated on deviations from the mean
of the evoked potential epoch (Buchsbaum 1976). This is obtained
from the amplitude values of the evoked potential by first subtract-
ng the mean of all values from each individual value and then
calculating the mean of those coordinates between 76 and 112 msec,
using each number as a positive value (absolute value). This
echnique also yielded the highest intraclass correlations in across
win pairs (except for the single point at 100 msec). Peak-to-trough
amplitude/intensity slopes had lower reliabilities ($r = .52$) and
measures based on a prestimulus baseline were noticeably unreli-
able. While it might be argued that an increase in the components
such as P300 might markedly raise the mean level of the evoked
potential, thus contaminating the P100 measure, this is rarely the
case. Without an assigned task, late components are not so large
and tend to return to baseline by 400–450 msec; inclusion of the
prestimulus 32 msec period also appears to anchor the evoked
potential baseline.

Multivariate techniques using amplitude at fixed latencies have
been used to yield reliable amplitude/intensity slopes for auditory
evoked potentials (Schachter et al. 1976). An empirical computer
algorithim method for peak identification based on examining
evoked potentials at multiple intensities appears to yield relatively
high test-retest reliabilities for identification of component latencies
but no test-retest reliabilities for amplitude/intensity slopes are reported (Hall et al. 1973*b*).

Evoked Potential Augmenting/Reducing Reliability

As indicated in the preceding section, reliability depends at least
partly on the reliability of the evoked potential component measurement technique. Reliabilities of the visual evoked potential measure
of augmenting/reducing are given in Table 31. Reliabilities for
various measures of auditory evoked potential amplitude intensity
functions are given in Schachter et al. (1976). Shagass and Schwartz
(1963) report test-retest reliabilities of .82 for somatosensory evoked

TABLE 31

TEST-RETEST RELIABILITY OF EVOKED POTENTIAL AUGMENTING/
REDUCING FOR P100–N140 MSEC COMPONENT

Author	Technique	Test-Retest Correlation
Buchsbaum and Pfefferbaum 1971	Peak-trough, normals	.71
Buchsbaum et al. 1971	Peak-trough, patients	.67
Buchsbaum 1974	Peak-trough, twins	.52
Buchsbaum 1974	Absolute area relative to mean, 76–112 msec	.63
Soskis and Shagass 1974	Area integral 75–150 msec	.54
Stark and Norton 1974	Peak-trough	.72

potential amplitude/intensity slopes in early evoked potential components.

Evoked Potential Reducing, Pain Tolerance, and Sensory Sensitivity

Like perceptual approach reducing, evoked potential reducing appears to be associated with pain tolerance and analgesia. We studied 32 normal college students who were divided into groups of pain tolerant and pain intolerant on the basis of a psychophysical procedure (Buchsbaum 1975). Examination of somatosensory evoked potentials, recorded very much like the visual evoked potentials, demonstrated the pain tolerant group to be evoked potential reducers (Fig. 36). Similar results were obtained using visual evoked potentials (Knorring et al. 1974). In this study, affective disorder patients were divided into evoked potential augmenters and reducers, and the reducers showed significantly higher electric shock pain thresholds and tolerance levels. Knorring (1975) also reported that patients with depressive disorders who reported pain complaints were significantly more likely to be visual evoked potential augmenters. Not entirely consistent results were reported by Mushin and Levy (1974), who found 25 patients suffering from psychogenic pain to have lower amplitude/intensity slopes. These results were based on very early somatosensory evoked potential components (N20–P30) so that the direction of the finding is not

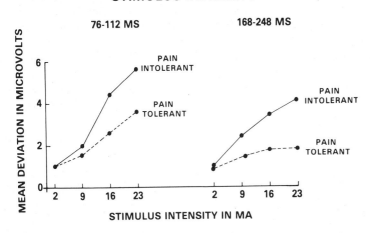

Fig. 36. Mean somatosensory evoked potential amplitude for four intensities of electric shock for the 76–112 msec and 168–248 msec time bands (generally equivalent to P100 and P200). Subjects were divided into pain-tolerant and -intolerant groups on the basis of their subjective ratings of shock unpleasantness. Pain-tolerant subjects are relative reducers—have lower rates of increase in evoked potential amplitude with increasing stimulus intensity.

clearly comparable. A component-by-component analysis of pain tolerance and evoked potential relationships is needed to fully resolve this issue.

Analgesia has also been associated with evoked potential reducing. Lavine et al. (1976) found that both subjective rating responses and somatosensory evoked potential amplitude/intensity slopes for P100 decreased during loud music paired with the suggestion of audioanalgesia. Sitaram et al. (1977) found P100 amplitude significantly diminished by physostigmine, which also decreased subjective pain judgments.

At the low end of the intensity scale, reducers appear to have larger evoked potentials (Silverman et al. 1969). This suggested that enhanced sensory sensitivity might create a compensatory need for reduction at high intensity levels. The loss of reducing, at least for auditory evoked potentials, during stages 3 and 4 of sleep is also consistent with an active inhibitory process in certain individuals (Buchsbaum et al. 1975).

Animal Studies

One of the possible advantages of evoked potential measurements of augmenting/reducing is the opening of a wedge into the almost impossible problem of the neurophysiology of personality by permitting animal studies. The ability to record from specific central structures as well as to stimulate specific inhibitory pathways is essential to understanding the underlying mechanisms. Hall et al. (1970) made observations of cats' exploratory, aggressive, and sensory response behavior, and also recorded evoked potentials to four intensities of light. Cats with high ratings for activity, aggressiveness, and exploratory behavior were augmenters whereas reducer cats showed low ratings. Lukas and Siegel (1977) confirmed these findings in evoked potentials recorded from the visual cortex in paralyzed cats with immobilized pupils, previously rated behaviorally. They extended these findings by demonstrating that reducer cats' cortical responsiveness decreased following all intensities of reticular stimulation whereas cortical responsiveness in the augmenters was at control levels or above. Thalamic responses showed no such individual differences. These findings seem to indicate that evoked potential augmenting/reducing occurs cortically and may be related to the interaction of ascending visual signals with brain stem arousal mechanisms. These authors also draw attention to an important aspect of neurophysiology traditionally overlooked—that individual animals may have quite different cortical response patterns and that these differences can be explored experimentally rather than be ignored or explained as an exception to the rule.

*Clinical Groups and Evoked Potential
Augmenting/Reducing*

Clinical group differences are summarized in Table 32. Reviews of the detailed psychophysiology of evoked potential augmenting/reducing (Buchsbaum 1975, 1977) and of its psychiatric correlates (Silverman 1972; Buchsbaum 1975) have appeared elsewhere. Perhaps the most robust and thoroughly investigated clinical correlate of augmenting has been its association with bipolar affective illness (often termed manic-depressive psychosis). We have reported off-medication bipolar patients to be evoked potential augmenters in two studies at NIMH (Buchsbaum et al. 1971, 1973). We also found bipolar patients to be augmenters on somatosensory evoked potentials (Buchsbaum 1977). In studies of affective patients in Israel (Gershon and Buchsbaum 1977) and of psychotic patients (Borge 1973), augmenting was also observed. Lithium, a common pharma-

TABLE 32

CLINICAL CORRELATES OF EVOKED POTENTIAL AUGMENTING/REDUCING

CORRELATES FOR AUGMENTERS	REFERENCES
Bipolar affective illness	Buchsbaum, Landau, Murphy, and Goodwin (1973)
	Buchsbaum, Post, and Bunney (1972)
	Gershon and Buchsbaum (1977)
	Milstein, Small, Moore, and Corsaro (1973)
Psychotic depressives	Borge (1973)
Paranoid schizophrenics	Inderbitzen, Buchsbaum, and Silverman (1970)
Neurotic patients with affective disorders	Knorring, Espvall, and Perris (1974)
Acting-out adolescents	Silverman, Buchsbaum, and Stierlin (1973)
Down's syndrome	Gliddon, Busk, and Galbraith (1975)
Alcoholics	Coger, Dymond, Serafetinides, Lowenstam, and Pearson (1976)
	Knorring (1976)
Alcoholics having relatives with bipolar affective illness	Martin, Becker, and Buffington (1977)
Normal women, children	Buchsbaum, Henkin, and Christiansen (1974)

CORRELATES FOR REDUCERS	REFERENCES
Acute schizophrenics	Landau, Buchsbaum, Carpenter, Strauss, and Sacks (1975)
	Rappaport, Hopkins, Hall, Belleza, and Hall (1975)
	Schooler, Buchsbaum, and Carpenter (1976)
Pseudohypoparathyroidism	Buchsbaum, King, and Henkin (1972)
Insomniacs (auditory evoked potentials)	Coursey, Frankel, and Buchsbaum (1975)
Unipolar affective illness	Buchsbaum, Landau, Murphy, and Goodwin (1973)
Normal men, older individuals	Buchsbaum, Henkin, and Christiansen (1974)

cological treatment for mania, was found to produce reducing (Buchsbaum et al. 1971), and further, augmenters were found more likely to show clinical response to lithium (Buchsbaum et al. 1971; Baron et al. 1975). Augmenting has been found in alcoholics (Knorring 1976; Coger et al. 1976), in relatives of patients with affective illness (Gershon and Buchsbaum 1977), and in alcoholics with relatives with affective illness (Martin et al. 1977). Evoked potential augmenting also appears associated with high scores on the Sensation Seeking Scale (Zuckerman et al. 1974), which has been correlated with hypomania, drug use, and other features possibly related to bipolar affective illness. Ludwig et al. (1977) noted that alcoholics who were augmenters were more likely to work for and consume alcohol.

Augmenting was also examined in a population of individuals potentially at risk for psychiatric disorders. This population was identified by screening 375 college student volunteers for low platelet monoamine oxidase (MAO) activity, an abnormality previously reported in bipolar affective and schizophrenic patients (Buchsbaum et al. 1976). Families of male low probands had an eight-fold increase in the incidence of suicide or suicide attempts over the incidence in families of high MAO probands; all probands with such a history were augmenters themselves. In a sample of 79 off-medication psychiatric patients, male individuals with evoked potential augmenting and low MAO showed a significantly higher incidence of suicide attempts than non-augmenting patients with either low or high MAO (Buchsbaum et al.1977).

Among acute schizophrenics, reducing seems more common (Landau et al. 1975; Shagass 1973). Reducer schizophrenics appear to be more likely to improve during hospitalization (Landau et al. 1975), suggesting perhaps some protective function. This reducing observed in schizophrenics seems consistent with the general tendency for smaller evoked potentials in schizophrenics, especially when stimuli are more intense, close together, novel, or uncertain— all stimulus aspects which might lead to sensory overload (see Buchsbaum 1977 for review). From a neurochemical viewpoint, it is interesting that Gottfries et al. (1976) noted evoked potential reducers among 26 psychiatric patients to have higher levels of homovanillic acid in their cerebrospinal fluid—indicative of higher dopamine turnover and generally consistent with the dopamine biochemical hypotheses of schizophrenia.

Most studies which relate evoked potential augmenting/reducing and drug action have been carried out in psychiatric patients, and thus the issues involved are beyond the scope of this survey. These include studies of amphetamine in hyperactive children (Buchsbaum and Wender 1973; Hall et al. 1970), phenothiazines in schizophrenics (Rappaport et al. 1975), and lithium in affective disorder patients (Buchsbaum et al. 1977). Normal subjects given depressants (pentobarbitol and ethyl alcohol [Spilker and Callaway 1969]) or tobacco (Hall et al. 1973a) both showed reducing, although the evoked potential techniques were somewhat different. A series of pharmacological studies in normal individuals with component-by-component analysis will be helpful in understanding evoked potential augmenting.

References

ARMINGTON, J. C., 1976a, "Adaptational changes in the human electroretinogram and occipital response," *Vision Research* 4:179–92.

———, 1964b, "Relations between electroretinograms and occipital potentials elicited by flickering stimuli," *Documenta Ophthalmologica* 18:194–206.

ATKINSON, W. H., 1976, "Electrophysiological evidence for Stevens' power law at the medial geniculate of the cat," *Brain Research* 109:175–78.

BARNES, G. E., 1976, "Individual differences in perceptual reactance: A review of the stimulus intensity modulation individual difference dimension," *Canadian Psychological Review* 17:29–52.

BARON, M., GERSHON, E. S., RUDY, V., JONAS, W. Z., and BUCHSBAUM, M. S., 1975, "Lithium response in depression as predicted by unipolar/bipolar illness, average evoked response, COMT and family history," *Arch. Gen. Psychiat.* 32:1107–11.

BLACKER, K. H., JONES, R. T., STONE, G. C., and PFEFFERBAUM, A., 1968, "Chronic users of LSD: The acidheads," *Am. J. Psychiat.* 125:97–107.

BORGE, G. F., 1973, "Perceptual modulation and variability in psychiatric patients," *Arch. Gen. Psychiat.* 29:760–63.

BUCHSBAUM, M. S., 1974, "Average evoked response and stimulus intensity in identical and fraternal twins," *Physiological Psychology* 2:365–70.

———, 1975, "Average evoked response augmenting/reducing in schizophrenia and affective disorders," in *Biology of the major psychoses: A comparative analysis*, edited by D. X. Freedman (Raven Press, New York).

———, 1976, "Self-regulation of stimulus intensity: Augmenting/reducing and the average evoked response," in *Consciousness and self-regulation*, edited by G. E. Schwartz and D. Shapiro (Plenum Press, New York).

———, 1977, "The middle evoked response components and schizophrenia," *Schizophrenia Bulletin* 3:93–104.

————, forthcoming, "The average evoked response technique in the differentiation of bipolar, unipolar and schizophrenic disorders," in *Psychiatric diagnosis: Exploration of biological criteria*, edited by H. Akiskal (Spectrum, New York).

BUCHSBAUM, M. S., COURSEY, R. D., and MURPHY, D. L., 1976, "The biochemical high risk paradigm: Behavioral and familial correlates of low platelet monoamine oxidase activity," *Science* 194:339–41.

BUCHSBAUM, M. S., GILLIN, J. C., and PFEFFERBAUM, A., 1975, "Effect of sleep stage and stimulus intensity on auditory average evoked responses," *Psychophysiology* 12:707–12.

BUCHSBAUM, M. S., GOODWIN, F., MURPHY, D. L, and BORGE, G., 1971, "AER in affective disorders," *Am. J. Psychiat.* 128:19–25.

BUCHSBAUM, M. S., HAIER, R. J., and MURPHY, D. L., 1977, "Suicide attempts, platelet monoamine oxidase, and the average evoked response," *Acta Psychiat. Scand.* 56:69–79.

BUCHSBAUM, M. S., HENKIN, R. I., and CHRISTIANSEN, R. L., 1974, "Age and sex differences in averaged evoked responses in a normal population with observations on patients with gonadal dysgenesis," *Electroencephalogr. Clin. Neurophysiol.* 37:137–44.

BUCHSBAUM, M. S., KING, C., and HENKIN, R. I., 1972, "Average evoked responses and psychophysical performance in patients with pseudohypoparathyroidism," *J. Neurol. Neurosurg. and Psychiatry* 35:270–76.

BUCHSBAUM, M. S., LANDAU, S., MURPHY, D. L., and GOODWIN, F., 1973, "Average evoked response in bipolar and unipolar affective disorders: Relationship to sex, age of onset, and monoamine oxidase," *Biol. Psychiatry* 7:199–212.

BUCHSBAUM, M. S., and PFEFFERBAUM, A., 1971, "Individual differences in stimulus intensity response," *Psychophysiology* 8:600–611.

BUCHSBAUM, M. S., POST, R. M., and BUNNEY, W. E., JR., 1977, "AER in a rapidly cycling manic-depressive patient," *Biological Psychiatry* 12:83–99.

BUCHSBAUM, M. S., and SILVERMAN, J., 1968, "Stimulus intensity control and the cortical evoked response," *Psychosomatic Medicine* 30:12–22.

BUCHSBAUM, M. S., VAN KAMMEN, D. P., and MURPHY, D. L., 1977, "Individual differences in AER to D- and L-amphetamine with and without lithium carbonate in depressed patients," *Psychopharmacology* 51:129–35.

BUCHSBAUM, M. S., and WENDER, P., 1973, "Average evoked responses in normal and minimally brain dysfunctioned children treated with amphetamine," *Arch. Gen Psychiat.* 29:764–70.

CLYNES, M., KOHN, M., and LIFSHITZ, K., 1964, "Dynamics and spatial behavior of light evoked potentials, their modification under hypnosis, and on-line correlation in relation to rhythmic components," *Ann. N. Y. Acad. Science* 112:468–509.

COGER, R. W., DYMOND, A. M., SERAFETINIDES, E. A., LOWENSTAM, I., and PEARSON, D., 1976, "Alcoholism: Averaged visual evoked response amplitude-intensity slope and symmetry in withdrawal," *Biological Psychiatry* 11:435-43.

COPPOLA, R., 1977, "A table-driven system for stimulus-response experiments," *Proc. of the Digital Equipment Users Soc.* 3:1219-22.

COURSEY, R. D., BUCHSBAUM, M. S., and FRANKEL, B. L., 1975, "Personality measures and evoked responses in chronic insomniacs," *J. Abn. Psychiat.* 84:239-49.

DEVOE, R. G., RIPPS, H., and VAUGHAN, H. G., 1968, "Cortical responses to stimulation of the human fovea," *Vision Research* 8:135-47.

DUSTMAN, R. E., and BECK, E. C., 1965, "The visually evoked potential in twins," *Electroencephalogr. Clin. Neurophysiol.* 19:570-75.

GERSHON, E. S., and BUCHSBAUM, M. S., 1977, "A gentic study of average evoked response augmentation/reduction in affective disorders," in *Psychopathology and brain dysfunction*, edited by C. Shagass, S. Gershon, and A. J. Friedhoff (Raven Press, New York).

GOTTFRIES, C. G., KNORRING, L. VON, and PERRIS, C., 1976, "Neurophysiological measures related to levels of 5-hydroxyindoleacetic acid, homovanillic acid, and tryptophan in cerebrospinal fluid of psychiatric patients," *Neuropsychobiology* 2:1-8.

HALL, R. A., GRIFFIN, R. B., MOYER, L., HOPKINS, H. K., and RAPPAPORT, M., 1976, "Evoked potential, stimulus intensity, and drug treatment in hyperkinesis," *Psychophysiology* 13:405-18.

HALL, R. A., RAPPAPORT, M., HOPKINS, H. K., and GRIFFIN, R. B., 1970, "Evoked response and behavior in cats," *Science* 170:998-1000.

———, 1973a, "Tobacco and the evoked potential," *Science* 180:212-14.

———, 1973b, "Peak identification in visual evoked potentials," *Psychophysiology* 10:52-60.

INDERBITZEN, L. B., BUCHSBAUM, M. S., and SILVERMAN, J., 1970, "EEG-averaged evoked response and perceptual variability in schizophrenics," *Arch. Gen. Psychiat.* 23:438-44.

KNORRING, L. VON., 1975, "The experience of pain in depressed patients: A clinical and experimental study," *Neuropsychobiology* 1:155-65.

———, 1976, "Visual averaged evoked responses in patients suffering from alcoholism," *Neuropsychobiology* 2:233-38.

KNORRING, L. VON, ESPVALL, M., and PERRIS, C., 1974, "Averaged evoked responses, pain measures, and personality variables in patients with depressive disorders," *Acta Psychiat. Scand. Suppl.* 255:99-108.

KOOI, K. A., and BAGCHI, B. K., 1964, "Observations on early components of the visual evoked response and occipital rhythms," *Electroencephalogr. Clin. Neurophysiol.* 17:638-43.

LANDAU, S. G., BUCHSBAUM, M. S., CARPENTER, W., STRAUSS, J., and SACKS, M., 1975, "Schizophrenia and stimulus intensity control," *Arch. Gen. Psychiat.* 32:1239-45.

LAVINE, R., BUCHSBAUM, M. S., and PONCY, M., 1976, "Auditory analgesia: Somatosensory evoked response and subjective pain rating assessment," *Psychophysiology* 13:140-48.

LEWIS, E. G., BECK, E. C., and DUSTMAN, R. E., 1972, "The evoked response of monozygotic, dizygotic, and unrelated individuals: A comparative study," *Electroencephalogr. Clin. Neurophysiol.* 30:162.

LUDWIG, A. R., CAIN, R. B., and WILKER, A., 1977, "Stimulus intensity modulation and alcohol consumption," *Quar. Journal of Alcohol.* 38:2049.

LUKAS, J. H., and SIEGEL, J., 1977, "Cortical mechanisms producing evoked potential augmenting-reducing in cats," *Science* 198:73.

MARTIN, D. C. BECKER, J., and BUFFINGTON, V., forthcoming, "An evoked potential study of endogenous affective disorders in alcoholics," in *Evoked brain potentials and behavior,* edited by H. Begleiter (Plenum Press, New York).

MILSTEIN, V., SMALL, J. G., SMALL, I. F., and SHARPLEY, P., 1975, "Evoked potential augmenting and reducing in psychiatric patients," abstracted, *Electroencephalogr. Clin. Neurophysiol.* 38:544.

MUSHIN, J., and LEVY, R., 1974, "Averaged evoked response in patients with psychogenic pain," *Psychol. Med.* 4:19-27.

PETRIE, A., 1974, "Reduction or augmentation? Why we need two 'planks' before deciding," *Percept. Mot. Skills* 39:460-62.

PICTON, T. W., GOODMAN, W. S., and BRYCE, D. P., 1970, "Amplitude of evoked responses to tones of high intensity," *Acta Otolaryngol.* 70:77-82.

RAPPAPORT, M., HOPKINS, H. K., HALL, K., BELLEZA, T., and HALL, R. A., 1975, "Schizophrenia and evoked potentials: Maximum amplitude, frequency of peaks, variability, and phenothizaine effects," *Psychophysiology* 12:196-207.

RICHEY, E. T., KOOI, K. A., and WAGGONER, R. W., 1966, "Visually evoked responses in migraine," *Electroencephalogr. Clin. Neurophysiol.* 21:23-27.

RIETVELD, W. J., 1963, "The occipitocortical response to light flashes in man," *Acta Physiol. Pharmacol. Neerl.* 12:373-407.

RIETVELD, W. J., and TORDOIR, W. E. M., 1965, "The influence of flash intensity upon the visual evoked response in the human cortex," *Acta Physiol. Pharmacol. Neerl.* 13:160-70.

RUST, J., 1975, "Genetic effects in the cortical auditory evoked potential: A twin study," *Electroencephalogr. Clin. Neurophysiol.* 39:321-28.

SCHACHTER, J., LACHIN, J. M., KERR, J. L., and WIMBERLY, F. C., 1976, "Measurement of electroencephalographic evoked response: Comparison of univariate and multivariate," *Psychophysiology* 13:261-68.

SCHOOLER, C., BUCHSBAUM, M. S., and CARPENTER, W. T., 1976, "Evoked response and kinesthetic measures of augmenting/reducing in schizophrenics: Replications and extensions," *J. Nerv. Ment. Dis.* 163:221-32.

SHAGASS, C., 1973, "Evoked response studies of central excitability in psychiatric disorders," in *AER and their conditioning in normal subjects and psychiatric patients*, edited by A. Fessard and G. LeLord (Inserm, Paris).

SHAGASS, C., and SCHWARTZ, M., 1963, "Cerebral responsiveness in psychiatric patients," *Arch. Gen. Psychiat.* 8:87-99.

SHAGASS, C., SCHWARTZ, M., and KRISHNAMOORTI, S., 1965, "Some Psychologic correlates of cerebral responses evoked by light flash," *J. Psychosom. Res.* 9:223-31.

SHIPLEY, T., JONES, R. W., and FRY, A., 1966, "Intensity and the evoked occipitogram in man," *Vision Research* 6:657-67.

SILVERMAN, J., 1972, "Stimulus intensity modulation and psychological dis-ease," *Psychopharmacologia* 24:42-80.

SILVERMAN, J., BUCHSBAUM, M. S., and HENKIN, R., 1969, "Stimulus sensitivity and stimulus intensity control," *Percept. Mot. Skills* 28:71-78.

SITARAM, N., BUCHSBAUM, M. S., and GILLIN, J. C., 1977, "Physostigmine analgesia and somatosensory evoked responses in man," *Eur. J. Pharmacol.* 42:285-90.

SOSKIS, D. A., and SHAGASS, C., 1974, "Evoked potential tests of augmenting-reducing," *Psychophysiology* 11:175-90.

SPILKER, B., and CALLAWAY, E., 1969a "Effects of drugs on 'Augmenting/Reducing' in averaged visual evoked responses in man," *Psychopharmacologia* 15:116-21.

————, 1969b, "'Augmenting' and 'Reducing' in averaged visual evoked responses to sine wave light," *Psychophysiology* 6:49-57.

STARK, L. H., and NORTON, J. C., 1974, "The relative reliability of AER parameters," *Psychophysiology* 11:600-602.

VAUGHAN, H. G., and HULL, R. C., 1965, "Functional relation between stimulus intensity and photically evoked cerebral response in man," *Nature* 206:720-22.

WOOTEN, B. R., 1972, "Photopic and scoptopic contributions to the human visually evoked cortical potential," *Vision Research* 12:1647-60.

ZUCKERMAN, M., MURTAUGH, T., and SIEGEL, J., 1974, "Sensation seeking and cortical augmenting-reducing," *Psychophysiology* 11:535-42.

BIBLIOGRAPHY

ADRIAN, E. D., 1928a, *Basis of sensation* (Norton, New York).
————, 1928b, *The basis of sensation: The action of sense organs* (Christophers, London).
BEECHER, H. K., 1959, *Measurement of subjective responses* (Oxford Univ. Press, New York).
BEXTON, W. H., HERON, W., and SCOTT, T. H. 1954, "Effects of decreased variation in the sensory environment," *Canad. J. Psychol.* 8:70–76.
BISHOP, G. H., 1959, "The relation between nerve fiber size and sensory modality: Phylogenetic implications of the afferent innervation of cortex," *J. Nervous Mental Disease* 128:89–114.
BLOUGH, D. S., 1958, "New test for tranquilizers," *Science* 127:586–87.
BORING, E. G., 1950, *A history of experimental psychology* (Appleton-Century-Crofts, Inc., New York).
BRILL, H., 1961, personal communication.
BYRON, G. N. G., 1899, Letter to Miss Milbanks (later Lady Byron) dated September 6, 1813, in *The works of Lord Byron; Letters and Journals III,* edited by G. E. Prothero (London), p. 400.
CARLIN, S., DIXON WARD, W., GERSHON, A., and INGRAHAM, R., 1962, "Sound stimulation and its effect on dental sensation threshold," *Science* 138:1258–59.
CARRIGAN, P. M., 1960, "Extraversion-introversion as a dimension of personality: A reappraisal," *Psychol. Bull.* 57:329–60.

CHERTOK, L., 1959, *Psychosomatic methods in painless childbirth* (Pergamon Press, New York).

COHEN, L. D., KIPNIS, D., KUNKLE, E. C., and KUBZANSKY, P. E., 1955, "Case Report: Observations of a person with congenital insensitivity to pain," *J. Abnorm. Soc. Psychol.* 51:333.

DALLENBACH, K. M., 1939, "Pain: History and present status," *Amer. J. Psychol.* 52:331–47.

EYSENCK, H. J., 1955, "Cortical inhibition, figural aftereffects, and theory of personality," *J. Abnorm. Soc. Psychol.* 51:94–106.

———, 1957, *The dynamics of anxiety and hysteria* (Routledge and Kegan Paul, London; Praeger, New York).

———, 1959, *The Maudsley personality inventory* (British Ed. Univ. London Press, Ltd. United States Ed., 1962; manual by Robert R. Knapp, Educational and Industrial Testing Service, San Diego).

———, 1960, *The structure of human personality,* 2d ed. (Methuen, London).

———, supv., 1962, *A report on personality factors and smoking,* part 2 (prepared by Mass-Observation, Ltd.).

EYSENCK, H. J., TARRANT, M., WOOLF, M., and ENGLAND, L., 1960, "Smoking and personality," *Brit. Med. J.* 1:1456–60.

FRANK, C. M., 1961, "Conditioning and abnormal behavior," *Handbook of abnormal psychology,* edited by H. J. Eysenck (Basic Books, Inc., New York).

FREEMAN, W., and WATTS, J. W., 1950, *Psychosurgery in the treatment of mental disorders and intractable pain* (Thomas, Springfield, Ill.).

GARDNER, W. J., LICKLIDER, J. C. R., and WEISZ, A. Z., 1960, "Suppression of pain by sound," *Science* 132:31–32.

GERARD, R. W., 1951, "The physiology of Pain: Abnormal neuron states in causalgia and related phenomena," *Anesthesiology* 12:1–13.

GIBSON, J. J., 1933, "Adaptation, after-effect and contrast in the perception of curved lines," *J. Exper. Psychol.* 16:1–31.

GREEN, G., 1951, *The end of the affair* (Bantam Books, New York).

HAENSZEL, W., SHIMKIN, M. B., and MILLER, H. P., 1956, "Tobacco smoking patterns in the United States," in *Public Health Monog.* No. 45 (U.S. Dept. of Health, Education, and Welfare, Public Health Service, Washington).

160   Bibliography

HARDY, J. D., WOLFF, H. G., and GOODELL, H., 1952, *Pain sensations and reactions* (Williams and Wilkins, Baltimore).

HEAD, H., 1920, *Studies in neurology* (Kegan Paul, London).

HEATH, C., 1958, "Differences between smokers and non-smokers," *AMA Arch. Intern. Med.* 101:377–88.

HEBB, D. O., 1949, *The organization of behavior* (Wiley, New York).

HENKIN, R. I., GILL, JR., J. R., and BARTTER, F. C., 1963, "Studies on taste thresholds in normal man and in patients with adrenal cortical insufficiency: The role of adrenal cortical steroids and of serum sodium concentration," *J. Clin. Invest.* 42:727–35.

HENKIN, R. I., DALY, R. L. and OJEMANN, G. A., 1967, "On the action of steroid hormones on the central nervous system in man," *J. Clin. Invest.* (in press).

JENSEN, A. R., "The Maudsley personality inventory," in *Sixth Mental Measurements Yearbook,* edited by O. K. Buros (in press).

KEELE, K. D., 1957, *Anatomies of pain* (Blackwell, Oxford).

KLEIN, G. S., and KRECH, D., 1952, "Cortical conductivity in the brain injured," *J. Pers.* 21:118–48.

KÖHLER, W., and DINNERSTEIN, D., 1947, "Figural after effects in kinesthesis," in *Miscellanea Psychologica,* edited by A. Michotte (Joseph Vrin, Paris), pp. 196–220.

KÖHLER, W., and WALLACH, H., 1944, "Figural after-effects," *Proc. Am. Phil. Soc.* 88:269–357.

LILLY, J. C., 1956, "Mental effects of reduction of ordinary levels of physical stimuli on intact healthy persons," *Psychiat. Res. Reports* 5:1–28.

LIVINGSTON, W. K., 1943, *Pain mechanisms* (Macmillan, New York).

MATARAZZO, J. D., and SASLOW, G., 1960, "Psychological and related characteristics of smokers and non-smokers," *Psychol. Bull.* 57:493–513.

MCARTHUR, C., WALDRON, E., and DICKINSON, J., 1958, "The psychology of smoking," *J. Abnorm. Soc. Psychol.* 56:267–75.

MELZACK, R., and SCOTT, T. H., 1957, "The effect of early experience on the response to pain," *J. Comp. Physiol. Psychol.,* 50:155–161.

MELZACK, R., and WALL, P. D., 1965, "Pain mechanisms: A new theory," *Science* 150:971.

MICHAELS, J. J., 1955, *Disorders of character* (Thomas, Springfield, Ill.).

MORAVIA, A., 1961, *The empty canvas* (La Noia). (Farrar, Straus and Cudahy, New York).

NAFE, J. P., 1934, "The pressure, pain and temperature senses," in *Handbook of general experimental psychology,* edited by C. Murchison (Clark Univ. Press, Worcester, Mass.).

NEISSER, U., 1959, "Temperature thresholds for cutaneous pain," *J. App. Physiol.* 14:368–72.

NISSEN, H. W., CHOW, K. L., and SEMMES, J., 1951, "Effects of restricted opportunity for tactual, kinesthetic, and manipulative experience on behavior of chimpanzee," *Amer. J. Psychol.* 64:485–507.

NOORDENBOS, W., 1959, *Pain* (Elsevier, Amsterdam).

PETRIE, A., 1952, *Personality and the frontal lobes* (Blakiston, New York. La Prensa Medica Mexicana, Mexico City. Routledge and Kegan Paul, London).

———, 1958, "Effects of chlorpromazine and of brain lesions on personality," in *Psychopharmacology,* edited by H. D. Pennes (Harper, New York) pp. 99–115.

———, 1960, "Some psychological aspects of pain and the relief of suffering," *Ann. N. Y. Acad. Sci.,* 86:13–27.

PETRIE, A., and COLLINS, W., 1960, "Perceptual differences as related to the tolerance of pain and suffering," *Proc. XVIth Int. Cong. Psychol., Bonn.* and *Acta Psychol.,* 29:755–56.

PETRIE, A., COLLINS, W., and SOLOMON, P., 1958, "Pain sensitivity, sensory deprivation and susceptibility to satiation," *Science,* 128:1431–33.

———, 1960, "The tolerance for pain and for sensory deprivation," *Amer. J. Psychol.* 73:80–90.

PETRIE, A., HOLLAND, T., and WOLK, I., 1963, "Sensory stimulation causing subdued experience—audio-analgesia and perceptual augmentation and reduction," *J. Nervous and Mental Disease,* 127:312–21.

PETRIE, A., McCULLOCH, R., and KAZDIN, P., 1962. "The perceptual characteristics of juvenile delinquents," *J. Nervous and Mental Disease,* 134:415–21.

POSER, E., 1960, "Figural after-effect as a personality correlate," *Proceedings of the XVIth International Congress of Psychology*

(North Holland Publishing Company, Amsterdam), p. 748–49.

QUADFASSEL, F. A., 1957, personal communication.

REES, G., 1960, *A bundle of sensation* (Chatto and Windus, London).

ROTHMAN, B. T., 1964, *Sensory augmentation.* Ph.D. thesis, Univ. Ottawa, Ottawa, Canada.

RYAN, E. D., and FOSTER, R., 1967, "Athletic participation and perceptual reduction and augmentation," *J. of Personality and Social Psychol.* (in press).

RYAN, E. D., and KOVACIC, C. R., 1966, "Pain tolerance and athletic participation," *Perceptual and motor skills* 22:383–90.

SCHONFIELD, J., 1966, personal communication.

SCHREIBER, W. S., 1962, personal communication.

SILVERMAN, J., 1964, "Perceptual control of stimulus intensity in paranoid and non-paranoid schizophrenia," *J. Nervous and Mental Disease,* 139:545–549.

———, 1966, "Variations in 'cognitive control' and psychophysiological defense in the schizophrenics," *Psychosomatic Medicine* (in press).

SOLOMON, P., KUBZANSKI, P. E., LEIDERMAN, P. H., MENDELSON, J. H., TRUMBULL, R., and WEXLER, D. (eds.), 1961, *Sensory deprivation* (Harvard Univ. Press, Cambridge, Mass.).

SOLON, J. A., 1967, manuscript to be published.

SPITZ, H. H., and LIPMAN, R. S., 1960, "Reliability and intercorrelation of individual differences on visual and kinesthetic figural after-effects," *Percept. Motor Skills* 10:159–66.

STONE, L. J., and DALLENBACH, K. M., 1934, "Adaptation to the pain of radiant heat," *Amer. J. Psychol.,* 46:229–242.

TRAVELL, J., 1959, personal communication.

WEBER, E. H., 1851, "Der Tatsinn und das Gemeingefühl," in *Handwörterbuch der Physiologie,* edited by R. Wagner (Vieweg, Braunschweig, Germany), Vol. 3, Pt. 2.

WEBSTER, 1959, *New World Dictionary of the American Language.* College ed. (World Publishing Co., Cleveland and New York).

WEDDELL, G., 1955, "Somesthesis and the chemical senses," *Ann. Rev. Psychol.,* 6:119–136.

WERTHEIMER, M., 1955, "Figural after-effect as a measure of metabolic efficiency," *J. Pers.* 24:56–73.

WERTHEIMER, M., and WERTHEIMER, N., 1954, "A metabolic interpretation of individual differences in figural after-effects," *Psychol. Rev.* 61:279–80.

WHITE, J. C., and SWEET, W. H., 1955, *Pain, its mechanisms and neurosurgical control* (Thomas, Springfield, Ill.).

WOLFF, B. B., and JARVIK, M. E., 1964, "Relationship between superficial and deep somatic threshold of pain with a note on handedness," *Amer. J. Psychol.,* 77:589–99.

Index